The His and Her's
GUIDE TO
Pregnancy
and Birth

The His and Hers GUIDE TO Pregnancy and Birth

DEAN AND STEPH BEAUMONT

Vermilion

LONDON

1 3 5 7 9 10 8 6 4 2

Vermilion, an imprint of Ebury Publishing,
20 Vauxhall Bridge Road,
London SW1V 2SA

Vermilion is part of the Penguin Random House group of companies whose
addresses can be found at global.penguinrandomhouse.com

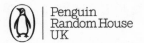

Copyright © Dean Beaumont and Steph Beaumont, 2016

Dean Beaumont and Steph Beaumont have asserted their right to be
identified as the authors of this Work in accordance with the Copyright,
Designs and Patents Act 1988

First published in the United Kingdom by Vermilion in 2016

www.penguin.co.uk

A CIP catalogue record for this book is available from the British Library

ISBN 9781785040368

Printed and bound in Great Britain by Clays Ltd, St Ives PLC

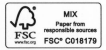

Penguin Random House is committed to a
sustainable future for our business, our readers
and our planet. This book is made from Forest
Stewardship Council® certified paper.

Dedication

This book is dedicated to our four amazing children:

Oren and Willow, whose pregnancies and births were the original inspiration for the approach, support and classes developed under The Natal Family.

Brock and Heath, who gave us the gift of two empowering and positive births and babymoons, while still showing us that in parenthood, there will always be something new to learn or experience.

Contents

Introduction

Congratulations! Whether you are actively trying to get pregnant and have bought this book to be super-prepared, or are already part way through your pregnancy experience, this is your guide to the journey of pregnancy and birth.

The *His and Hers Guide to Pregnancy and Birth* will take you through each part of this experience, both from your individual perspectives as mum and dad, as well as together as a partnership. Along the way you are likely to find that you both have different thoughts, roles and concerns, and this guide aims to help you both prepare and navigate your individual paths, while bringing you together as a parenting team.

So who are we? We are Dean and Steph Beaumont, leading antenatal educators in the UK, who also happen to be husband and wife with four children between us!

Dean was the UK's first male professional antenatal educator, and is the founder of the innovative, award-winning antenatal education programme for dads, DaddyNatal. His first book *The Expectant Dad's Handbook* was published by Vermilion in 2013.

Steph is an antenatal educator who has worked with thousands of parents to prepare for birth. She is the founder of MummyNatal, a birth preparation programme that empowers women to understand more about their birthing bodies and have the confidence to make their own birth choices.

The birth of our first child eight years ago was a life-changing moment in more ways than one. The birth was difficult and we were both left feeling as though the antenatal classes we had attended had not prepared us for what occurred during labour and birth; we felt we had been given little understanding of what was happening and how to manage.

We came to realise that there was a lack of good, unbiased support for parents preparing to have a baby, and this inspired us to retrain and change careers to become antenatal professionals.

For over six years, as well as teaching separately, we have worked together to co-teach couples antenatal workshops, unique in that they are co-facilitated by both female and male professional antenatal educators. Our workshops and approach treat *both* parents as integral in the pregnancy and birth; they are about bringing a couple together to prepare for and welcome their baby, and recognise each role for its importance and value.

Our workshops explain how mums and dads will experience parts of the journey through the pregnancy and birth differently, and why. Men and women are different, and understanding what is going on in the mind of your partner is a unique and important aspect of our approach; it allows for increased understanding, and less stress and fewer arguments!

We both wished that we had been able to attend this sort of workshop at the time of the birth of our children. We never seemed to understand where the other was coming from, and we started to recognise a pattern of disagreements between us, as well as between friends who were also expecting! As we started teaching, we would often get asked the question: 'Is it just us who argue about x?' or 'Is it just us who can't agree on y?' – and the answer was always no; many couples experience the same misunderstandings, which we hear about all the time, but unless you know that, it can feel like you are the only people going through these issues. It seemed obvious to us that making couples aware that these things are common and why they occur, might lead to less stress. And less stress when you are pregnant or have a new baby to care for, has got to be a good thing!

As not all parents can access one of our workshops, and as our family continues to grow, it is harder for us to teach together. We have also had many women contact us to say that they read their partner's copy of *The Expectant Dads Handbook* and loved it, and wanted something they could read too. So, we put all of this together and decided that, even seven years after we started our couples' classes, there is still an information gap for parents. While there are many books out there aimed at mums or dads, we couldn't find a comprehensive, single book which caters for both mum *and* dad together.

Since you have created a baby together and will be parenting him or her together, it makes sense that you may also want to prepare for that together. So here it is, the *His and Hers Guide to Pregnancy and Birth*, aiming to support you both with everything you need to know to prepare for the birth of your baby.

Getting Started

This book is split into three main sections: Pre-conception, Pregnancy, and Labour and Birth. The pregnancy section is divided into stages and months. We suggest reading each chapter at the beginning of the relevant month in your pregnancy. This will help guide you through the choices, tools and information for each stage.

In case your baby is born a little earlier than you are expecting, we would suggest making sure you have been able to both read through the Labour and Birth section by 35 weeks of pregnancy. You can read these sections at any time (and you are likely to want to go through them a few times), although there are also little signposts as you read through the pregnancy section to suggest when to dip into these sections.

You will see that each chapter follows a similar structure:

- a *Hers* section for mum to read
- a *His* section for dad to read
- a *Get Together* section, which is for you both to read, and suggests key choices or preparations that you may both want to think about.

Of course, it is also perfectly fine to read the section written for your partner, especially if you want to gain more insight into what he or she might be experiencing and going through.

The approach we take is that becoming parents is easiest done if you approach it as a team. It is about learning to look out for each other, and accepting that you both have different roles to play which you will do in your own ways, which when you put them together makes for a fantastic partnership. We hope that you find that the *His and Hers Guide to Pregnancy and Birth* helps you to achieve this.

section one

The journey begins

CHAPTER 1

Trying for a baby

If you are not yet pregnant but are hoping to be soon, here are our tips on how to conceive. We also explain about pregnancy testing and go through all the lingo you will encounter on the way.

Hers

During your menstrual cycle, your eggs mature in your ovaries until hormonal changes cause one (or more) eggs to be released; this is known as ovulation. Ovulation usually happens about 14 days after the first day of your last period, although it does vary. This released egg travels into one of your fallopian tubes.

To become pregnant naturally, your egg needs to meet your partner's sperm in your fallopian tube. Your egg will live for about 12–24 hours after it's released, so to get pregnant, a sperm must fertilise the egg within this time.

You are most likely to get pregnant if you have sex within a day or so of ovulation. However, sperm can survive for up to seven days inside your body after sexual intercourse, which means that an egg can be fertilised by sperm that entered the body before the egg was released.

When trying for a baby, some couples choose to just carry on with their normal sex life and wait to see what happens. Others choose to try and increase their odds of getting pregnant by working out when ovulation occurs and by making sure they have sex around this time.

Although learning about when you ovulate is interesting and might make you feel more in control of your baby-making efforts, studies show that regular sex, every 2–3 days throughout your cycle gives you the best chance of conceiving.

There are various ways to try and work out when you are ovulating. Look for signs of hormonal and physical changes in your body that signal ovulation is about to occur:

■ **Notice any changes in your cervical mucus.** This is the vaginal discharge that you notice when you go to the toilet. As you become fertile, your cervical mucus changes to become clear, slippery and stretchy, a bit like raw egg whites. This is to support the sperm's journey to your egg, by making it easier to swim through.

■ **You can chart your basal body temperature (BBT).** To record your BBT, you will need to use a basal thermometer which has a finer scale than a normal thermometer. When you ovulate, hormonal changes trigger a tiny rise in your BBT. It take can take a few cycles to be able to recognise your individual pattern, and you need to take your temperature first thing each day for the results to be valid.

■ **You can use an ovulation calendar.** This will help you to try and predict when you are likely to ovulate. Although ovulation tends to be around day 14 of each cycle, this is not the case for every woman. You can literally use your own diary to keep track of your cycles and likely fertile periods, or download an app for your phone which will work that out for you from the data you put in.

■ **You can use an ovulation testing kit**. These are urine tests which look for luteinising hormone (LH) and can help you to track when you are most fertile. When the LH is at its highest, it triggers an egg to release, so your testing kit can show you when that is about to happen.

In couples with no fertility difficulties, there is a 20–25 per cent chance of getting pregnant during each cycle. It is worth knowing that 80 per cent of women, who are under 40 and having regular sex without using contraception, will get pregnant within a year. If it hasn't happened this month, if doesn't mean it won't next month, so don't give up hope if it doesn't happen right away. It can be difficult to hear about someone becoming pregnant when you are trying to conceive yourself, but remember that it has no bearing on your odds.

Pregnancy testing

To get the most reliable result with a pregnancy test, you take it on the day you expect your period to start. Home pregnancy tests are very accurate when used according to their instructions; they work by testing for the presence of hormone human chorionic gonadotrophin (HCG) in your urine.

Some women find that they have the urge to repeatedly test to see if they get a positive; if you find that you want to test regularly you are not alone! Many women are so keen to get pregnant that they test more regularly than is needed; if you test too early the HCG may not be strong enough to be picked up by a pregnancy test, so you may get false negatives. The amount of HCG doubles in your body every 48 hours, so if you get a negative in the morning, you are unlikely to get a different result later that day.

Trying to conceive jargon

There are lots of online groups and forums for women who are trying to conceive. The abbreviations that they sometimes use can be off-putting at first: '*We BD-ed when I got the go ahead from the OPK and CM looked good, but getting through the TWW is so hard for a POAS addict like me! I want to know whether it's a BFP or I'm awaiting AF again!*' The jargon can be quickly learnt though if you want to get involved, and here is a quick lowdown of some essential terms:

DTD: Doing the deed (sex)

BD-ing: Baby dancing (also means sex!)

CM: Cervical mucus

OPK: Ovulation predictor kit

POAS: Pee on a stick (pregnancy testing)

TTC: Trying to conceive

AF: Aunt Flo (period/menstruation)

BFN: Big fat negative (not pregnant on a pregnancy test)

BFP: Big fat positive (pregnant on a pregnancy test)

DPO: Days past ovulation (generally need to wait 14 of these for testing)

FMU: First morning urine (using this for a pregnancy test as it has the most concentrated hormones)

TWW: Two week wait (the two weeks between ovulation and being able to do a pregnancy test)

His

Different couples approach trying for a baby in different ways. Your approach may depend on how long you have been trying to conceive, as well as your individual personality types. Sometimes men and women approach the idea of trying to conceive quite differently; for some men it can just be about not using contraception any more and seeing what happens, while the female partner might want a more proactive approach.

If you decide to try for a baby, discuss with your partner how you both want to approach it; there is no right or wrong, but knowing how you want to make it happen can help keep you both on the same page.

Your partner may use ovulation kits to try and maximise the chances of conceiving, or be looking out for physical signs that she is about to ovulate. The idea is that your partner knows when she is most fertile so can suggest you have sex on those days. Some men have told us that they can feel a little off put by having to have sex by the diary rather than spontaneously, feeling that it is clinical or forced. If you feel this way, talk to your partner and work out a way that you can both compromise.

It will vary from woman to woman, and may depend on how long you have been trying to conceive, but you might notice that your partner gets progressively more upset each month that she doesn't become pregnant. The anticipation which builds in the two weeks leading up to being able to take a pregnancy test, can be a time when hopes are really built up. If the test is negative, or her period arrives, it can be incredibly disappointing, especially if she thought she had been experiencing early pregnancy symptoms. If you notice that your partner is getting down each month, reassure her that you will keep trying. You could ask when her next period is due, so you know when she will be testing, and can offer to be there with her when she takes the test.

Get Together

Whehen you decide that you want to try for a baby, you can be surprised at how much it can take over your lives together. If sex becomes completely focused on trying for a baby, it can be easy to forget that you are also a couple who love each other. Continuing to make time for each other is important, and of course, can also improve your odds of conceiving!

Scheduling your sex life around a diary can create stress and can cause couples to want less sex. It's pretty obvious that if you are having sex less often, your chances of conceiving are smaller.

Stress may also inhibit conception because of its impact on the hypothalamus which regulates the production of hormones. In women it controls the hormones that cause the release of eggs, meaning that stress can also affect the menstrual cycle, causing changes in ovulation or even preventing ovulation. In men, it regulates their testosterone levels, which are responsible for both the production of sperm and libido, meaning that stress can lead to a lower sperm count, and a lack of interest or arousal for sex.

Reducing stress as a couple

If you are planning to get pregnant, why not discuss together how you can keep the stress low and enhance your bond as a couple, to minimise the likelihood? You know each other best as a couple, so sit and discuss what appeals to you and how you are going to take care of your relationship while trying for a baby.

- **Film night.** Get any essential chores out of the way and make time for a film night in. Share a bottle of wine, some good snacks and snuggle together on the sofa to have a night at the home movies.

- **Enjoy a meal together.** Book dinner out at a special restaurant, or cook something a little more special than your usual evening grub; set the table with candles and get dressed up. If it's warm enough, you could alternatively head out for a picnic.

- **Go to a spa together**. Enjoy a day of treatments and relaxation. If that's too much for the bank, why not share a bath together and give each other a massage?

- **Have a holiday.** We are often at our most relaxed when on holiday, which can help bring all the body chemistry into balance. So why not have a break away together, or even a weekend away and just see what happens?

- **Take the afternoon off.** Go for a walk in a beautiful place, or take a bike ride together.

CHAPTER 2

Unexpectedly expecting

If you have found yourself unexpectedly expecting, rest assured that you are not the first couple to have found yourself in this position. It will have no bearing on what kind of parents you will be, or how much you will love your baby.

The first few days and weeks can feel tumultuous as you both come to terms with the new direction your lives are taking, as you are undertaking a life change, with what feels like no preparation or choice. But be assured that some time to come to terms with it, and supporting each other as you adapt to the news, will make a huge difference.

Hers

Sometimes pregnancy is a surprise. Sometimes we find ourselves pregnant at a time in life when it would not have been our choice to be.

If you find yourself to be unexpectedly expecting, know that this is different from the pregnancy being a 'mistake' or it being 'unwanted'. It is important to recognise this distinction so you don't get overwhelmed by what you think you 'should' feel or what you 'should' do at a potentially vulnerable time.

How do you feel?

Surprise pregnancies are often accompanied by a range of emotions, including disbelief, anger, joy, fear, panic, excitement, guilt, embarrassment, happiness, shame or resentment.

It is not unusual to be conflicted about how you feel. Perhaps the pregnancy is a wonderful surprise and you are delighted about it, but are scared to tell your partner as you are worried he will not be. Maybe you are pregnant and don't want to be, but you think your partner will be over-the-moon. Sometimes surprise pregnancies are tricky because we know that we may not be on the same page as our other half.

It's not unusual for either or both of you to feel a sense of anger or resentment towards the baby, or just to feel disconnected from it. You may feel guilty at thoughts you have had, such as secretly hoping for a miscarriage, or wishing you weren't pregnant while knowing friends or family who desperately want to be. Feelings of obligation due to religious or moral beliefs can also come into the mix.

Maybe you feel as though you have 'messed up' in some way, and blame yourself. There is a widespread assumption that unplanned pregnancies are something which only happens to those who are immature or reckless, but this is not the case, and there are many more surprise pregnancies each year than people may think. Many people who find themselves unexpectedly pregnant don't always tell the world that's what has happened! Birth control can sometimes be unsuccessful – whether it is due to having a tummy upset while on the pill or missing a feed while breastfeeding; there are reasons why sometimes the measures we take to prevent pregnancy do not work. We are human, and sometimes we just take risks which do have consequences.

You might be fearful about what others will think or say when they find out, and whether they will judge or criticise your relationship, your circumstances, or your ability to raise a child. The list of possible reasons for having a bundle of mixed-up feelings is a long one, and thousands of people have been there before.

The good thing about pregnancy is that you get several months to adjust to the idea of having a baby, so try not to put too much emphasis on any confused feelings you may have in the first few days or weeks. Once the initial shock has subsided, most women (and their partners) do go on to form a bond and connection with their baby, as they would with any planned pregnancy.

So what do I do?

When you first find out about the pregnancy, you might find it helpful to get some emotional support. If your partner is not the first person you want to talk to and tell, that's okay. Just find someone to confide in who you know will be able to listen non-judgementally and who allows you to work through your thoughts and feelings. In an ideal world, your family and friends would be an obvious source of emotional support, but they may not be if you think they will feel conflicted or disloyal to your partner, or if they have strong opinions. A trusted friend, or even someone entirely separate from your life such as a counsellor, might give you a listening ear and non-judgmental support while you work things out.

When you do feel ready, find a time to sit down and talk to your partner. Prepare yourself for his possible shocked reaction; you have had an informational and emotional head start on him, and he may need some time to work through his thoughts and feelings too. Try not to take any immediate reactions to heart, and give him some time to let the news sink in. Be firm about how you feel though; you are the one carrying the baby and your feelings and preferences matter.

His

Finding out that you have made a baby when you were not planning to, it goes without saying, is one of the biggest surprises you can have in life.

Maybe you feel delighted at the news but your partner isn't, as she isn't feeling ready for a baby (or another baby) at this point in her life. Or maybe you didn't want a baby (or another baby) and you feel frustrated that there is now one on the way, as though your feelings have been ignored.

It is not unusual on the discovery of a pregnancy, even when it is planned, for one of you to have the thought: 'Am I ready?' or even, 'I'm not ready!' If you have experienced this, then you are not alone. At some point, the majority of all expectant dads have had this thought cross their mind, and yet still go on to be great fathers. These kinds of thoughts just mean that you are aware of the enormity of it all – and it could be argued, this awareness means you will make a fantastic dad!

Having a baby is always a huge life change, and it is completely normal to have one of those 'what have I done?!' moments! This is just what your brain does before any major life event, and they don't come much more major than this.

While these feelings and thoughts are normal, it is also important to understand where they come from and that they are often temporary. This allows you to think about how you respond to these thoughts and feelings, and how you communicate them with your partner.

However you feel about the situation, one thing to take a moment to consider is how difficult it had been for your partner to have found out about the pregnancy and tell you about it, especially if she knows you don't both feel the same way about it. She will have had lots of different thoughts and feelings too, and has had to face those in the same way you are having to, in addition to having to pluck up the nerve to tell you, not knowing how you will react. If you are reading this after having found out about a surprise pregnancy, think about how you reacted to the news.

If you are reading this, knowing that you have reacted in a way that has upset your partner, it is not too late to reassure or repair. Take the opportunity to apologise for your reaction and to acknowledge you understand she has valid feelings too; this can make a big difference to your relationship.

Get Together

How each couple responds to the news of an unexpected positive pregnancy test differs massively. After the initial shock wears off, you may both be overjoyed and quickly start planning the future with your new baby. Or, in some cases, you may still not be able to envisage life with a baby. Maybe you feel completely differently from each other.

However you both feel, there will be a lot of thoughts and feelings to process in the early days in order to move forwards with the pregnancy.

It can be helpful to separate how you feel from how you think you 'should' feel. You will not be the first parents who are not immediately excited about a new baby. Try not to judge yourselves as being 'bad' parents or people because of this – it doesn't mean that at all.

Be prepared that when you first find out it can all feel very intense and pressured. Give yourselves time to absorb the news; try to avoid making any decisions when either of you feels stressed or upset – leave the discussion and come back to it the next day when you both feel calmer and thinking is clearer. Likewise, don't make any decisions in the middle of the night – notoriously things always seem worse when we are exhausted.

When you discuss the pregnancy, try to focus on the future rather than the past, and avoid the 'blame game' – blaming each other, or yourself. Blame doesn't change anything and just continues to stir up negative feelings.

Focus on how you both feel and how you want to move forwards, rather than worrying about others around you. You are the two people who matter, and you are the two people who need to keep communicating. It can be hard enough to do this in periods of stress or worry, without also complicating it with worries about what other people might think. The opinion of your friends and family is not as important as it might first seem. If, when they find out about the pregnancy, they are not supportive to start with, that's okay; it's not their life or their pregnancy.

It sounds simple, but try to take it one day at a time. Give yourselves some time for the initial shock to subside, support each other, and keep talking.

section two

Pregnancy

CHAPTER 3

Congratulations! Month One

Congratulations on your pregnancy! The strange thing is that for the majority of the first month, you do not know you are pregnant yet! However, there is a lot which is going on at the point, so keep reading to find out more…

Hers

That positive pregnancy test can make women react in really different ways. Have you taken one test and got a positive result you feel satisfied with? Or are you still taking tests to check the result is the same? Neither reaction is unusual, so either way you are not alone! If you have seen a positive result within the time frame given on the instructions (usually between two and 10 minutes), even if the indicator is extremely faint, the test is likely to be positive. Home pregnancy tests are very accurate, and 'false positives' are very rare. If you want to be sure you are interpreting the test correctly, you can wait a couple of days and take the test again. You might find it helpful to use one of the digital tests on the market which will actually say 'pregnant' or 'not pregnant'.

How do you feel?

Getting that positive test can bring with it many feelings and emotions. Whether your baby was planned or not, the moment it becomes 'real' can bring up all kinds of thoughts and feelings which you might not expect.

There is often an expectation that pregnancy will flick a switch in a woman's brain, which turns her into a blooming, full-of-the-joys, happy, devoted earth goddess! For some women, this does happen and everything changes the moment they know. But for others this isn't the case, and that's normal too.

The only thing that is certain about pregnancy, is that every pregnancy is different. Every woman has different feelings, different symptoms and different experiences. While we might know this logically, it is still not unusual to have expectations of how we think we will feel (or 'should' feel). You may feel:

- Excitement and happiness, and want to immediately tell the world your news.
- Anxiety, thinking about the impact that a child will have on you and your family, and how it will change and affect your life.
- Guilt or concern about things you have done in the days/ weeks before getting the positive pregnancy test, such as having had an alcoholic drink.
- Anxiety about something going wrong during the pregnancy.
- Guilty if not immediately bouncing with joy, thinking that negative thoughts mean you do not love the baby enough, and are therefore somehow not good enough.
- You might start happily daydreaming about your little one, about who he or she will look like, and be like.
- You might be keen to plan how soon you can take maternity leave and whether you want to go back to work or become a stay at home mum.

- You might not feel anything! Some people feel quite numb and unsure of how they feel. Staring at the test; putting it away and then getting it out to look at it again; double-checking the line; weeing on another one to check it was right – these are all normal reactions too.

'We had been trying for a baby for a few months, but when we got that positive test result I remember thinking: "What have we done?! We aren't ready!" Those feelings went away though, and we had a great pregnancy and loved becoming parents. When we got pregnant the second time and the same thoughts came up again, I worried a lot less about them as I knew they weren't real!' – **Hannah**

case study

Be reassured that any of these thoughts, and many possible others, are completely normal! Any thoughts we perceive to be 'negative' do not make us a lesser parent or inadequate. Just because we think something, does not mean it is true; it's just a thought. The brain creates all these thoughts and feelings as part of the process of interpreting and processing information. Planned or not, the confirmation of a pregnancy is life-changing information, and when it changes from an idea to being real (like any other life changing event) it is normal to feel lots of different things!

Women often don't feel they can admit to any feelings which are less than joyful, because we are 'not supposed' to feel these things, so they are often kept secret. This is slightly bonkers of course, as there are so many women having them! The basic truth is that these feelings are not a reflection of how much you love your baby or how good a parent you'll be. What the worry and anxiety actually shows is that you do care, and that you do recognise how big and important what you are about to do is. It just shows how much you *are* prepared for the realities of becoming a parent!

Pregnancy symptoms

Physically, what can you expect to feel at this point in your pregnancy? Pregnancy symptoms can be a bit misleading this early on, as some women will feel nothing at all, or you may just experience symptoms which are very similar to your usual menstruation aches and pains. Symptoms alone are usually not enough to predict if you are actually pregnant; you need to take a test. Although every pregnancy and pregnant woman is different, here are some of the early signs which you might notice:

- Tender breasts
- Light bleeding or spotting around the time that you usually have your period. This is called 'breakthrough bleeding'. It is perfectly normal, but it is always best to get any bleeding checked by your GP.
- Nausea or queasiness
- Not being able to stomach certain foods, drinks or even smells
- Spot breakouts
- Nothing at all. If you have no symptoms at all, this is also completely normal and is nothing to worry about!

Positive result, what do I do now?

- **Make a booking appointment with a midwife.** This can vary a little in different areas, but usually this can be done by calling your local GP's surgery. These appointments are usually held when you are about nine weeks pregnant (when you have missed two periods). However, if you have questions which you feel you need answers to before then, such as about medications you're currently taking, existing health conditions or any worrying symptoms, do go ahead and make an appointment with your GP or the community midwife.

- **Start to learn about pregnancy.** You can sign up online for a week-to-week guide to pregnancy – many of these will send you email updates telling you a little about what is happening with baby that week. You could also sign up for an early pregnancy class to help you prepare for some of the decisions you will have to make during pregnancy.

- **Be aware of your lifestyle.** Becoming pregnant does not mean that you have to completely change your lifestyle. If you are used to regular exercise such as jogging or swimming, there is no need to stop doing this, though you might like to get advice if you do a very physical sport. You could start to look at any changes you want to make for your pregnancy: eating a balanced diet, making time for some rest and relaxation, getting plenty of sleep – all these things will help you through your next few weeks of pregnancy, and even the birth.

- **Plan for anything which does urgently need to change.** If your work or workplace could affect the wellbeing of your pregnancy, you may wish to consider that as soon as possible. This is especially the case if you work with x-rays or chemicals, have a very manual job or one that puts you into situations where potentially you could be injured. Also think about anything in your personal life which might need some adjustments, such as travel plans and whether these will still be okay or how to accommodate them. Consider how you want to handle any social events or parties where you might be expected to drink or eat certain things which you wish to avoid, and how you want to handle that. A bit of creativity often solves many situations!

- **Take folic acid.** Folic acid is important for baby's development, as it can significantly reduce the risk of neural tube defects, such as spina bifida. The Department of Health recommends that women take a daily supplement of 400 micrograms of folic acid while trying to conceive, and should continue for the first 12 weeks of pregnancy, which is when a baby's spine is developing. If you didn't take folic acid supplements before getting pregnant, then you can start taking them as soon as you find out that you are.

- **Enjoy your pregnancy.** The first few days and weeks of pregnancy can be a very special time. Everything can still be a bit surreal before the real symptoms and appointments start to kick in, and even more so if no one else knows about it. It can feel like a very special, private secret, and having a meal out, or some non-alcoholic bubbles, or doing something similar which feels celebratory for you (but is also safe in pregnancy), is a nice way to welcome it in.

His

Congratulations, you have a baby on the way!
Maybe you were there and waited for the test result with your partner or maybe you have just been told the news. Either way, it is a big moment and there is bound to be quite a bit for you to get your head around.

How do you feel?

Just because you are not the one carrying the baby doesn't mean that pregnancy has no impact on you. Whether the pregnancy has been planned for months or years, or is unexpected, you are likely to feel a range of emotions at different points.

Both you and mum might be experiencing mixed feelings about the pregnancy and it is completely normal for both of you to feel like this. Becoming a parent is a life-changing event, and it is normal to feel anxious, excited, protective of your partner, increased joy and pride in the relationship and also in your ability to create a baby!

However old we are, and whatever life experiences we may have had to date, even if the pregnancy is something you have been looking forward to, the thought of not being sure if you are 'ready' is normal.

Sometimes you may experience underlying feelings of uncertainty, which may be expressed as crankiness towards your partner, wanting to spend more evenings out with your friends, or flirting with other women. These reactions are normal, but they are no help to your situation or partner who needs extra support at this time. Be aware if you notice any of these reactions occurring so you can handle them appropriately – knowing why they are happening is often the key for bringing them under control, and preventing them cause potential disagreements and problems.

Men are often 'fixers', and being aware of the desire is important. Male thoughts about pregnancy can quickly turn to become potential 'issues', and we can start planning to solve them, which can detract from enjoying the moment. That is not to say that making plans is not important; it is of course, but perhaps getting the calculator out to work out the implications on finances straight after the positive pregnancy test is not the best timing!

It's also natural to feel left-out sometimes. The changes that are taking place for your partner aren't always obvious, and naturally your partner's attention will be on what's happening to her and the baby. It can be the first sign that your relationship is changing to accommodate another person, and that can take a while to adjust to for both of you.

It is also completely normal to have days when you don't think about the pregnancy, or really have any feelings about it one way or another. For a lot of men, visual or physical signals are an important way of making it all 'real' for us, so it may not really sink in until you have heard a heartbeat or seen a scan.

How does she feel and what am I meant to do?

It is common for dads to feel that there isn't a great deal they can do – but this is just not true; your role as a dad starts now, in the way that your partner's role as mum has begun. In these early days, your role is what you can do to help with the changes that are taking place.

What is important to consider, is that, as you may be going through a host of different feelings and thoughts, so will she. Your partner has all the life-changing realities to deal with, as you do, and all the physical and hormonal changes that happen as part of pregnancy. This can affect how a woman feels from day-to-day, or even hour-to-hour. It can be difficult for you to predict how she is going to feel, and you do run the risk of doing or saying the wrong thing.

Just remember that this is all normal and part of pregnancy. Try to resist the urge to define what exactly is 'wrong', so you can fix it. Equally, just telling your partner 'not to worry' if something is bothering her is really not going to help either. Listen to her, and tell her you understand without trying to solve the 'problem'. All the mood swings and mixed-up feelings can be as unnerving for her as for you, and sometimes a hug and a sympathetic ear will make a big difference.

Get Together

*B*y four weeks into pregnancy, your baby is the size of a poppy
seed. The placenta and umbilical cord are in place to support
your baby's growth.

There will be lots of things which you might want to start discussing together at this point in the pregnancy; it is all part of processing the news and starting to prepare for the arrival. If you want to start discussing baby names, plans for the birth, or what colour to decorate the nursery, then go ahead and enjoy it. Having just found out the news, an obvious topic for discussion this month has to be:

When do we tell other people our news?
First up, this is your news as a couple, so it is useful to think through what feels right for you both. Agreeing on who you are going to tell/not tell and when can also save you both from potential disagreements in these early weeks.

Some people tell everyone right away, while others wait until they have had their first 'dating scan' at around 12 weeks.

There isn't a right or a wrong time to make your announcement, it is whatever feels right to you. These days most people seem to feel there is an expectation or moral obligation to wait until 12 weeks. Some women we have spoken to even feel judged if they announce before this point, as they have felt that others will see them as taking a 'risk' in doing so, and it is more 'appropriate' to wait for the nod from the medical establishment.

However, the first 12 weeks does not have to be a secret because it is more 'ladylike' or 'appropriate'. Announcing your news earlier will always be met with disapproval from some as it isn't the choice they would make, but this is *your* pregnancy. If it feels right for you, then that is what matters.

If you would prefer more privacy, then equally, 12 weeks is not an official time when an announcement 'should' be made. It is nobody's business but your own when you decide you wish to share *your* news.

It can be helpful to consider the implications of when you wish to announce, to help you make your decision. It will depend on what is important to you, and how the pregnancy goes in those first few weeks. As with many things in life, it can be useful to have a preference to work towards, but to be prepared to re-evaluate it if things are not quite as you expect!

If you decide to keep your pregnancy private until the dating scan (or beyond), this means that you are choosing to keep the first third (at least) of the pregnancy a secret. This means potentially not disclosing any early pregnancy symptoms. For some women who have only minor early pregnancy symptoms, this can be relatively straight forward. For some women, early pregnancy can be the most challenging part of the whole experience and having other people know can be helpful as they can get more support rather than feel they are suffering in silence

'In my pregnancy I was hospitalised with hyperemesis (severe vomiting). I still look back at that pregnancy and think about how more support from those around me might have helped, rather than keeping the pregnancy a secret until 12 weeks because that is what we "should" do.' – **Jenny**.

case study

The risk of miscarriage drops dramatically by the time of the dating scan, and this is often seen as a good reason for not sharing the news until then. Should you miscarry, you won't have to explain to the whole world and deal with ongoing difficult questions from people who may not have heard the sad news. However, it can also mean that if a miscarriage does happen, that there isn't the support and understanding around either. You may decide that a miscarriage will be easier to cope with, with fewer people knowing about it, and so privacy is the right decision for you. For couples who have had previous difficulties in early pregnancy, or are going through IVF treatment, then they may want privacy, or just the support of a few close friends and family. We all need and want different things.

Many parents will know that early pregnancy can be a time of mixed emotional feelings, and those of anxiety or worry are just as normal as the more 'positive' emotions. Keeping your news private while you come to terms with your feelings, or deciding to tell people so that you can talk about them are both options, and depend on what kind of person you are.

You may wish to tell a couple of important people early on and even wait to tell everyone else until it is evident to see! There are plenty of parents who don't tell anyone until the baby begins to make its existence obvious.

When weighing up your decision, try not to focus on what you 'should' do, or what your family or friends have done – think about what you *want* to do. You can always choose to keep it private and then change your minds later, but if you do this, try to remember that the decision to change your mind also needs to be done in agreement together, rather than one of you breaking the agreement you have made together!

How are you going to make your announcement?

There are lots of ways which people choose to make their announcements, and the popularity of social media has added a lot of variations too. Whether you decide to let the people who matter know face-to-face, or you want to make a big creative announcement to share on Facebook, or something else entirely, this is an exciting choice you can now make and plan together!

Here are some ideas, and searching the internet for 'pregnancy announcements' will give you a lot more!

- **Occasion cards.** Giving a birthday or Christmas card to 'Grandma', 'Granddad', 'Auntie' etc. from the baby, with a photo of the scan inside, is one way to make your announcement unforgettable for key family members.

- **Big sibling announcements.** If you have older children, getting one of them a t-shirt that says: 'I'm going to be a big brother/sister', or something similar, is a nice way to get them involved in the news. We did this for our fourth pregnancy announcement (pictured below!).

- **Sharing scan images.** Many parents choose to share the image of their first scan to announce the pregnancy – simple but effective.

- **Creative photography.** Some parents get creative with their announcement – a line-up of the family's shoes plus a pair of baby booties is just one of endless possibilities.

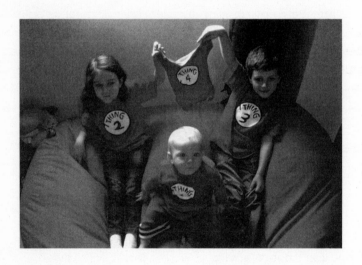

CHAPTER 4

Month Two

Your pregnancy begins to become real in lots of different possible ways this month, from early pregnancy symptoms, to lifestyle changes and the beginning of your antenatal care – it all begins here!

Hers

Pregnancy symptoms

If they haven't started already, this may be the month that early pregnancy symptoms appear, if you are going to experience them. Some women do not experience any symptoms, so if you don't notice anything, don't worry; every pregnancy is different, and you can have a perfectly healthy pregnancy with no symptoms at all.

If you do experience early pregnancy symptoms, most noticeably you may experience exhaustion and nausea. Nausea can be made worse by being tired, so get as much rest and sleep as you can to try and combat these symptoms. Tender breasts, a frequent need to urinate, skin breakouts and increased vaginal discharge are also all normal.

How do you feel?

It may all start to feel a little more real this month, as you start making arrangements and changes to your lifestyle now that the pregnancy has been confirmed.

Attending your first antenatal appointment can feel like a key milestone after the positive pregnancy test – it is normal to feel anxious and/or excited as towards the end of this month you may have, (or be getting ready for) your booking-in appointment, where your antenatal care begins.

You may also be considering your diet and anything you wish to cut down, cut out or introduce while you are pregnant. You don't need to go on a special diet, but it's important to eat a varied diet to get the right balance of nutrients that you and your baby need. If you find you are suffering with morning sickness, just focus on eating what you can keep down for now. Eating little amounts often can help with managing nausea, as hunger pangs can make it worse.

During pregnancy, it's important to make sure all fruits, salads and vegetables are washed thoroughly to remove any agricultural chemicals on them.

When it comes to diet, the official guidance to follow is:

- **Avoid soft blue cheese and soft cheeses with white rinds unless cooked.** This is because soft cheeses are less acidic than hard cheeses, and contain more moisture, which makes them a potential environment for harmful bacteria, such as listeria. Infection with listeria is rare, however, even a mild form of the illness can lead to miscarriage, stillbirth or severe illness in a new baby.

- **Hard cheeses are considered safe in pregnancy**. Even if made with unpasteurised milk, as bacteria are less likely to grow in hard cheese, so the risk is considered low.

- **Many soft cheeses are considered safe in pregnancy.** Cottage cheese, mozzarella, feta, cream cheese, paneer, ricotta, halloumi, goats' cheese and processed cheeses, such as cheese spreads are considered safe, as long as they are made from pasteurised milk (check the labels!).

- **Avoid all types of pâté**, including vegetable pâtés, as they can contain listeria.

- **Avoid raw or partially cooked eggs** or foods that contain raw and partially cooked eggs, such as homemade mayonnaise. This is to avoid the risk of salmonella. Salmonella food poisoning is unlikely to harm your baby, but it can give you a severe bout of diarrhoea and vomiting.

- **Avoid raw or undercooked meat** because of the potential risk of toxoplasmosis. Cook all meat and poultry thoroughly so it's steaming hot and there's no trace of pink or blood, especially with poultry, pork, sausages and minced meat, including burgers. Toxoplasmosis infection can damage your baby, but it's important to remember that toxoplasmosis in pregnancy is very rare.

- **Be cautious with cold cured meats.** Many cold meats, such as salami, Parma ham, chorizo and pepperoni are not cooked; they are just cured and fermented. This means that there's a risk of toxoplasmosis.

- **Avoid liver.** Liver or liver-containing products such as liver pâté, liver sausage or haggis, may contain a lot of vitamin A and too much vitamin A can harm your baby.

- **Fish is mostly safe to eat during pregnancy,** but you should avoid shark, swordfish and marlin because it contains more mercury than other types of fish, which in high quantities could affect your baby's developing nervous system. You should also limit the amount of tuna you eat, for the same reason.

- **Peanuts are safe** to eat during pregnancy, as recent studies show there is no link between the consumption of nuts and allergies, as was previously thought.

■ **Caffeine in pregnancy.** Regularly consuming more than the recommended amount of caffeine in pregnancy may increase the risk of miscarriage or a baby being born with a low birth weight. Caffeine is found in lots of foods, such as coffee, tea and chocolate, and is added to some soft drinks. You don't need to cut out caffeine completely, but the recommendation is to have no more than 200mg a day which is roughly equivalent to two mugs of tea or instant coffee a day, or one mug of filter coffee.

Booking appointment

Your booking appointment will take place at around 10 weeks of pregnancy. This is after you have missed two periods and the chances of miscarriage have decreased. To arrange a booking appointment call your local GP surgery.

The booking appointment is likely to be one of the longest antenatal appointments you will have – it can take around an hour. There is a lot of paperwork to complete, which will cover you and your partner's medical history, as well as your families'. You will also be asked:

■ **Date of your last period.** The midwife will work out an estimated due date, but also offer you a dating week scan at around 12 weeks, which he or she will use to determine a more accurate due date.

■ **Previous births, miscarriages and abortions**. The midwife will ask about previous pregnancies, births, the weight and stage of pregnancy any previous babies were born, and about any abortions, miscarriage or stillbirths.

■ **Medical history.** The midwife will ask about any medical conditions you have, or any which run in your or your partner's family; it is worth finding out about these before you go, if you don't know already. He or she will also ask about any complications or difficulties you might have experienced in a previous pregnancy.

- **Lifestyle.** You will be asked about the lifestyle of you and your partner, including whether you drink alcohol or smoke.

At this appointment, you will also be offered a check which involves taking your height and weight to calculate your BMI (body mass index); there are some increased risks to women who are classed as overweight, such as gestational diabetes and pre-eclampsia.

You will also be offered tests and checks which will become routinely carried out (if you consent for them to be) at each antenatal appointment from this point on. These include:

- **Antenatal urine tests.** At each antenatal appointment, the midwife can check your urine for several things, including the presence of protein. Sometimes a trace of protein can be found, and this is not usually a cause for concern, but it can be an indicator of an infection or pre-eclampsia, a condition which can be serious if not treated. You will be given a specimen bottle to collect a sample to bring to the next appointment.

- **Blood pressure monitoring.** Your blood pressure can also be routinely checked at every antenatal appointment. A rise in blood pressure, especially alongside the presence of protein in the urine and some other symptoms, can be a sign of preeclampsia.

His

These first months are a busy, busy time for your partner's body, as the baby manages to grow from just a single sperm and egg all the way up to the prawn-like character you see on the screen at the first scan. In addition, your partner grows an entire new organ – a placenta – to nour-ish the baby. All of this work can be exhausting, so if your partner is feeling fatigued at the moment, you now under-stand why. Support her to be able to rest when she needs to and understand that she might not feel able to be going on nights out or even staying up late to watch TV at this point.

Morning sickness might kick in with a vengeance this month. This is not as simple as just needing a puke in the morning – morning sickness can be all-day-long nausea, feel-ing similar to a hangover or even mild food poisoning. It can be very difficult to deal with, especially if your partner is still trying to keep the pregnancy a secret from work colleagues, and so trying to cope with feeling ill without letting anyone realise that she feels that way.

Tiredness can make nausea worse (so another reason to support her to rest when tired), as can the smells of some foods, so if your partner is the regular cook in your household, it might be time for you to take the chef role for a while.

The first few weeks can be a strange time for dads-to-be. As the changes taking place are not usually very visual, preg-nancy can feel a little unreal at this stage, and you may even find yourself completely forgetting about the pregnancy some days. This is quite normal.

Your partner has her first antenatal appointment at the end of this month, which you are welcome to attend with her. If you do go along, you should feel welcome – midwives should talk to you as well as your partner, and you should find two chairs put out when you attend appointments. The midwife is there to support you both, so if you have any questions, do ask them.

Get Together

B y week eight baby will be the size of a strawberry. Their arms and legs are lengthening and they are beginning to move around.

Around the end of this month is the booking appointment. This is the longest routine antenatal appointment you are likely to attend. It usually lasts about an hour, and occurs between weeks 8–12 of the pregnancy.

You will be asked where you want to birth your baby, so that the right paperwork can be completed; different hospitals have different sets of forms! Have a think beforehand about where you might choose. It is helpful to be aware that you are likely to have some of your antenatal care (scans and tests) done where you choose. You can change the place of birth later in the pregnancy if you wish; you do not have to give birth somewhere just because your antenatal care was there.

It's useful for you both to attend the booking appointment because there are questions about both of you and your medical histories. The answers help the antenatal team find out about any potential risks to mum or baby. You will be offered a dating scan, nuchal translucency scan, and blood tests, so you might want to discuss in advance which tests you wish to have and if there are any you wish to decline (see page 52). Remember though, you can always change your mind later if you wish about these too.

The appointment is also a great opportunity for either of you to ask any questions you may have, the midwife is there to support you both.

CHAPTER 5

Month Three

Going into the third month of your pregnancy, it can be a time of continued mixed feelings of nervous excitement, as you are offered a scan to check all is well with your baby. There are a lot of decisions which are yours for the making this month, so find out more and make time to discuss them together.

Hers

Pregnancy symptoms

As you come into the third month, you may be experiencing a raft of pregnancy symptoms. If you are going to experience the joys of morning sickness, it will have started by this point, but the good news is that, more often than not, nausea will start to ease by the end of this month. Every pregnancy is different though, and some women experience symptoms that last beyond 12 weeks, some women have no symptoms at all, and many women fall somewhere between. Try not to compare your symptoms with a previous pregnancy or with those a friend is having, as every pregnancy is different.

Your breasts may begin to get bigger and you might notice that some of your bras are not very comfortable any more. It can be a good time to consider getting measured for a supportive maternity bra, which can grow with you through pregnancy.

How do you feel?

You may find that your emotions vary greatly at this point: you may feel happy one moment and sad the next. Mixed emotions are normal but if you feel down a lot of the time, talk to your partner and mention it to your midwife.

A big milestone at around the end of the third month is the opportunity to have your dating scan, and this can come with a lot of emotional changes before, during and after. A lot of women look forward to this scan for reassurance, as it is (for many women) the first 'official' medical test which is done to confirm the pregnancy. Up until this point, everything has been based on your own tests and it isn't uncommon for us to wonder whether we have made a mistake. The scan can give that reassurance that it is all happening.

Seeing the form of your baby and their heartbeat is an exciting moment, whether it is your first or fifth; seeing that there really is a little person growing inside of you can be an awe-inspiring moment.

For a lot of women, we can feel a lot of anxiety as that scan date approaches. We might not even realise how much it is affecting us until the scan has passed and we suddenly feel the weight lifted away. Feeling on edge, depressed, crying or snapping at other people, and even an increase in nausea are normal reactions to any anxiety. For those women who find that their early pregnancy symptoms ease off at the end of this month, the lead up to a scan can lead to them coming back again! If you feel low, anxious or are experiencing mood swings, be assured that you are not alone.

The thing to bear in mind is that there is always something to worry about in any situation. We worry when we are puking ten times a day, because we worry that our baby might not be getting the nutrition they need to grow. We then worry when the puking stops because we think it means something has happened to our baby! We worry because we care, and to some extent that never goes away – we worry about the wellbeing of our children for the rest of our lives!

While very sad things do happen sometimes, for the vast majority of women, the 12-week scan shows that all is well. Try not to worry too much about all the things which could go wrong, and definitely don't sit up all night googling all the possibilities! As humans, we are naturally attracted to the negative; we retain the rare scary stories more readily than the more common positive ones, so avoiding looking at sad stories on the internet will help stop any anxiety going into overdrive.

If you notice that you are anxious, be kind to yourself in the few days leading up to the scan; don't take on anything crucial, or set too high expectations on what you should be achieving.

'I was absolutely bricking it about the 12-week scan. I was bursting into tears over every little thing in the couple of days beforehand, snapping at my other half all the time. On the way to the scan I felt so sick — I thought I'd just gotten up with really bad morning sickness, but as soon as we stepped in and saw a healthy little baby on the screen, all the sickness and anxiety just all went away. It was only then I realised how much I had been worrying that there was going to be a problem.' – **Erica**

case study

Your partner may be looking forward to the scan, or might come across as fairly apathetic. This point in the pregnancy can be difficult for men, as it can feel very unreal as there is not yet anything tangible for them to experience. The scan is often the point where it all starts to become more real for dads and they can catch up a little in terms of their feelings and thoughts. Bear in mind that if he doesn't appear overly excited before the scan, it isn't a reflection on how he feels about you or the baby.

What is the dating scan for?

Every pregnant woman in the UK is offered two routine scans, the first one is the 'dating scan' which is also known as the 12-week scan because of the time it is usually carried out in the pregnancy. However, try not to focus on '12-weeks' too much, as your scan might be arranged for slightly earlier or later than this; NICE (National Institute for Health and Care Excellence) recommends it is carried out between 10 weeks and 13 weeks. The scan is for a variety of things:

- **To confirm the pregnancy.** The sonographer will be looking for a baby (or more than one!) and their heartbeat/s.

- **You will be given an estimated due date (EDD).** This will be used throughout the rest of your pregnancy. This is calculated by measuring the baby from head to bottom, which is known as the 'crown rump length' (CRL). The EDD often differs to the date which you or the midwife may have worked out for yourself already, which was based on your last menstrual period (LMP).

What do I need to do before the scan?

You will usually have to drink quite a lot so you have a full bladder; the amount varies a little between hospitals, so check the appointment letter you have been sent to see what it suggests.

Drinking fluids for a scan can sound easier than done; timing is key! Drink your fluids too early and you may be bursting for the loo in the waiting room. If you are experiencing morning sickness or hyperemesis (see page 63), you may find drinking a lot difficult. Try sipping rather than gulping it down.

What happens during the scan?

The room will have a bed next to the scanning equipment, and is likely to be dimly lit for the scan to be easy to see. You will be asked to lie on your back on the bed, and to pull up your top to expose your tummy, and slightly pull down your trousers/skirt and knickers. If you want to avoid showing the sonographer your knickers in their full glory, don't wear a dress!

A gel will be squeezed onto your bump, followed by a handheld device moved over your lower abdomen. The sonographer will complete the observations and measurements, and put those in your notes. You can ask any questions you have. Most of the time, you will also be able to buy a scan photo to take home and keep as a memento; there may be a charge for this so take along some money.

His

This month you may notice that your partner is experiencing some challenging pregnancy symptoms. Morning sickness can be in full effect, so it can be a difficult time for your partner. Strong smells and tiredness can make nausea a lot worse, so try to give her as much opportunity to rest as possible and take over the cooking of the meals if that isn't your usual role (see page 36 for what she can and can't be eating).

A big milestone for this month is that you and your partner will be offered the first routine ultrasound scan. This scan checks everything is okay with your baby and will give you an estimated due date.

Ultrasounds only began to be used in the 1970s, and the technology behind them originates back to WWII and the detection of enemy submarines, before being adapted for medical use. Ultrasound scans use high frequency echoes from sound waves, which bounce off the baby and are translated into a computer image showing the baby's size, position and movement.

Most scans are carried out by specifically trained staff called sonographers. Your partner will be asked to lie down on a bed and to lower her skirt or trousers to the hips and raise her top so the sonographer can access her abdomen. The sonographer will put ultrasound gel on your partner's tummy and use a handheld device over the skin. It is this device that sends out the ultrasound waves and picks them up when they bounce back, translating them into a picture of your baby on the screen.

If you can attend the scan with your partner, there are lots of benefits for you both. In the UK, at time of publication, fathers have the right to take unpaid time off work to accompany their expectant partner, at up to two antenatal appointments, which include scans. However, some workplaces may give you much more flexibility than this to attend appointments, or indeed legislation may change, so always make sure you find out what you are entitled to. Using annual leave so you don't miss out on key appointments is also a choice you could make.

For dads, scans are a pretty awesome way to connect with your baby. Seeing your baby moving around and the little heart pumping away is an amazing moment. For many men, this is the first time it really hits home that you will be (or in fact ARE) a dad! A lot of dads say it is the first time it makes sense, or is when they feel a bond to their baby start to grow. Most places now offer you the opportunity to buy a scan photo to take home with you, so remember to take some money.

'I knew we were pregnant, but it didn't really compute until that first scan. Then it became very real for me. It was pretty amazing actually, which I hadn't expected. Seeing our baby on the screen and getting that scan photo meant it was really happening, and gave me something to focus on. I couldn't wait for the next scan!' – **Matt**

case study

The first scan can be exciting and nerve-wracking in equal measure for your other half – many women experience some anxiety that there 'might not be anything there'. If you notice your partner's mood or behaviour is a bit more stressed than usual on the day of the scan (or the days leading up to it), just be aware she may be worrying more than she is letting on or even realises herself. Just be as supportive as possible and keep reassuring her, if needed. Don't tell her to not worry or that she is being silly; her feelings are all part of her journey of becoming a mum. If you find she is scaring herself by reading things on the internet which are not helpful, try and distract or redirect her away.

The majority of the time, the scan is a really positive moment in a pregnancy. However, it is important to remember that it is a screening test, and occasionally will find a problem or raise a question. If this happens it can be distressing for you both, which is why supporting each other and being there if you can is so important.

If you cannot be there, discuss with your partner the option of someone else going with her for support. While the scan is a fantastic way of helping develop an early bond, it is certainly not the only way, so don't beat yourself up about it if you cannot attend. Instead, make sure that you get to see the scan photo, and find other ways to bond with your baby instead: listening to the heartbeat at a midwife appointment, going to the next scan, feeling the baby move (from about 24 weeks of pregnancy) or reading to the bump are other ways of supporting that bond to grow and for you to be involved.

Get Together

*B*y the end of this month, at around 12 weeks, your baby is tiny but fully formed. All of the organs, muscles, limbs and bones are in place, and although you won't be able to feel it yet, your baby is moving around!

One of the key choices you make together this month is about which tests you want to have. You will be offered a dating scan, and possibly also a nuchal translucency (NT) scan. These will have been mentioned at your booking appointment last month, but you always have the option to change your mind if you wish, right up until the moment of the scan, so it is worth thinking about at this stage too.

While the dating scan is usually an eagerly awaited part of pregnancy for the majority of parents, it is still important to know that it is a choice whether you have it done or not; it is not a requirement, and some parents choose not to have one. If you decide not to have this scan (or any scans), it will not affect you receiving any other antenatal care.

While scans are wonderful for bonding with baby, and have lots of positive aspects to them, it is also important to remember that they are medical tests.

Some parents-to-be want to find out if there are any concerns within the pregnancy, so they can be prepared and have options. Others feel that as any results won't change how they feel or their choice of actions, they don't need to know and therefore don't want them done. There is no right or wrong, just what feels right for you together.

When discussing what screening tests you wish to have, here are some of the key considerations:

Are there any risks with ultrasound scans?

There are no known risks of pregnancy ultrasound scans. However, this is not the same as saying they are proven to be safe. The easiest way to look at it, is that they have been widely used in medical practice for over 50 years, with no evidence of adverse side effects.

The small amount of waves that the baby is exposed to during a routine scan (which is usually quite short) is not thought to be enough to cause any damage. The diagnostic opportunity to identify any problems is thought to vastly outweigh the very small potential risk. However, this still ultimately remains your choice to weigh up together.

There is more uncertainty in the safety of ultrasounds for non-diagnostic reasons, such as for 3D photos or videos. These tend to require longer scans, which also have not been proven to be either safe or unsafe; it remains your decision to weigh up any risk.

Another risk for parents around the option of the scan, is the risk itself of discovering something (conclusive or not) which could cause you both distress and anxiety. Further tests may be offered as a result, which can carry their own risks. In some cases, it may transpire that there is nothing wrong with the baby and the distress caused was unnecessary.

What about the nuchal translucency (NT) scan?

In many areas of the UK you will be offered a nuchal translucency (NT) scan. This is usually carried out during your dating scan, and assesses how likely the risk is that your baby has Down's syndrome. During the scan, the pocket of fluid under the skin at the back of your baby's neck is measured; all babies have some fluid at the back of their neck, but often babies with Down's syndrome have more.

Because the NT scan involves taking this very specific measurement, it is possible to choose to have the dating scan but decline the NT scan. If you do this, the sonographer will just not take the NT measurement.

How accurate is the NT scan?

The NT scan will estimate how high or low the risk of your baby having Down's syndrome is – not whether they definitely do or don't. The results may say the baby is at high risk, but it is still possible they may not have Down's syndrome. Conversely, a baby could be shown to be at low risk, but it is still a small possibility they may have Down's syndrome. The only way to get a definitive result is to have an amniocentesis. A more invasive test, an amniocentesis comes with more risk, such as miscarriage, which is why it is not routinely offered to all women.

In addition, it is not always possible to obtain the NT measurement, as it depends on the position of the baby. If this is the case, you will be offered a different screening option.

So which tests should we have done?

Each test throughout the pregnancy will have its own perceived risks and benefits for you to weigh up together.

Many families decide to consent to all the tests offered so that they have as many options as possible and can be prepared if all is not well. This is absolutely fine and it is why the screening tests do exist and are offered to all.

However, some parents may not wish to have some, or any, of the tests, and this is your choice too.

The scans can sometimes lead to uncertainty, difficult decisions, and additional tests. If you do not want to take the risks of a diagnostic test to get a definitive answer, then it is important to consider together whether you wish to consent to a screening test which might raise the question.

The results of diagnostic tests could, in some instances, also lead to decisions about continuing or ending the pregnancy. These choices will always be your decision, and health professionals will support you whatever you decide – but it is likely to be a distressing time. If you wish to avoid having to make decisions like these, then it is worth bearing in mind which tests you consent to.

There is a balance between being able to enjoy all the exciting parts of an antenatal scan, with the understanding that testing for something means looking for problems. You can both feel assured that the vast majority of babies are healthy, and screening tests such as scans will just confirm that.

These are all very personal decisions to make, and so it is worth really discussing together what you both feel regarding what you want to know and when, and, if there is anything which you do not want to know or be tested for.

It's entirely up to you whether or not you have a dating scan or NT scan. You can always choose to have some tests and not others. You could have a dating scan without the NT screening, you could have the dating scan with the NT screening, or you could opt to have neither. You can make your final decision on the day of your scan, even if this is different from the decision you had previously made, and be supported with your decision.

Do your research, discuss the choices together, and decide what is right for you both.

CHAPTER 6

Month Four

This month marks a big milestone in your pregnancy, as once you have reached the end of week 13, you will now be into the second trimester! The great news is that the risk of miscarriage is now very low and you may start to notice that your early pregnancy symptoms, especially any morning sickness, are now starting to ease.

Hers

Your uterus has grown large enough to start to move up out of your pelvis and into the abdomen, which can lead to the beginnings of a 'baby bump'. Every woman's body is different, so you may feel that you are not showing at all, or that you are showing quite a lot – both are completely normal!

Pregnancy symptoms

Some other symptoms might kick in around now: it is not uncommon to experience some constipation as pregnancy hormones relax the bowel. You may also notice ligament pains and achy hips due to the hormone relaxin preparing your body for the birth (see page 63).

You may start to feel baby moving, although it is still very early and most first-time mums do not feel movements until around or after 20 weeks. At this stage movements are likely to feel like little bubbles popping in your abdomen, but as the weeks go by they become stronger and easier to distinguish as kicks.

How do you feel?

Pregnancy symptoms which you have been experiencing up until this point may still be present, but for many women things get easier this month, if they haven't already. Every pregnancy is individual, and things can change from one day to the next, so try not to feel despondent if you are not feeling the 'blooming' experience you have heard about – some women don't feel like this during pregnancy and it doesn't mean anything is wrong.

If you are feeling well at this point, you may find your sex drive is also back on track, or increased. It is safe to have sex during pregnancy (unless you have been specifically advised not to by a medical professional). However, if you do not feel in the mood, that is not uncommon either. Some women just have a lower sex drive when pregnant. However you feel, it is important to stay connected to your partner and to make sure he understands what is going on. Men look for affection to reassure that all is well in the relationship, and at a time of change (even happy change) this can be especially important to them. Making time for cuddles instead of sex and explaining how you feel will go a long way to reassure that there isn't a problem with him or your relationship.

Any early pregnancy signs, while not always pleasant, are a reassuring sign of the pregnancy, so it is not uncommon for women to have moments of worry about whether they really are still pregnant once those symptoms stop. Now you have reached this point in your pregnancy, the risks to your baby are much lower and it is most likely that everything is well. If you have concerns, you can always call your midwife to talk to him or her. It might be helpful to join a pregnancy class where you can meet other women and share experiences, which will also help you realise you are not alone in your thoughts. Why not look for a local aqua natal class or even join one of our mum-to-be MummyNatal classes, which will give you a bit of time to focus on your pregnancy, time to talk to other mums, and back up in a different way everything you are reading about in this book!

'I think of myself as quite a rational person, but during pregnancy I found myself worrying about everything. I worried when I had morning sickness that the baby wasn't getting the nutrients it needed, and I worried when the morning sickness stopped that it meant there was a problem with baby. Going to weekly classes where I met other mums going through the same thing helped put it into perspective and calmed me down.' – **Lindsey**

case study

His

The great news about the second trimester is that the risk of miscarriage reduces dramatically. The second trimester is known as the month when mum 'blooms' and has lots of energy – but be aware that this isn't always the case.

This month you may notice that your partner's pregnancy symptoms are beginning to change. It is helpful to be aware that as the symptoms ease off, some women feel anxious that this might signal a problem with the pregnancy. It is most likely everything is fine.

The widespread belief about the second trimester is that mum will suddenly feel full of energy and wellbeing, she will develop thick glossy hair and turn into a sex fiend ... sounds too good to be true? Yep, that's because these are all largely myths; pregnancies are individual and affect women in different ways. Just as some women find the first trimester difficult while others glide through without a symptom, some women experience lots of challenging symptoms in the second trimester while others feel fantastic. The only way you know how your partner is feeling, is by talking to her.

Alongside the 'pregnancy bloom' myth is another myth which can cause misunderstanding. Information for expectant dads often includes advice which tells us that women will go through changes to their sex drive during pregnancy e.g. first they go off sex, then they want it, and then they go off it again. Of course, this may be true for some women, as the hormone changes may affect them in this way, but this is not a general rule. How your partner feels about sex may change from day to day, or she may have a varying sex drive for the whole nine months.

Other aspects of the pregnancy will also influence how she feels about sex. In reality, Mum may well not feel in the mood if she is still spending most of her day feeling or being sick – this is pretty understandable!

The changes to your partner's body can feel deeply unattractive to her – larger tummy, stretchmarks, heartburn, reflux, sickness – none of these things are a recipe for feeing sexy. While to you, she may still look perfect, if she doesn't feel that way, it may well affect her libido. It is important that you understand this so that you don't take a low libido personally.

What if you are not in the mood? After all, it is not uncommon for men to experience a change of sex drive when (and after) their partner becomes pregnant.

For some of us, we cannot shake the thought that we might hurt the baby, or that it is 'inappropriate' now the baby is present! Once your partner looks pregnant, it can affect how you feel about sex, as it becomes a constant reminder that there is someone else involved.

You may have concerns about hurting your partner or the baby, or bringing on premature labour. While there are specific medical conditions when sex during pregnancy is not advised, these are the exception not the norm. If you should be avoiding sex you will be advised of this by your midwife or doctor. If you do find that your sex drive is lower than usual, talk to your partner about it, and find other ways to be affectionate instead.

As your partner's body shape changes, you will have to find positions in which you can both enjoy sex and accommodate the bump; it's part and parcel of having sex during pregnancy!

'I wasn't expecting my sex drive to change once Imogen became pregnant, but it did, especially once we had seen the baby on our scan and her bump started to show ... I felt very protective of her and our baby, and I think on some level I was worried that I might hurt them. ' – **David**

case study

Get Together

By the end of this month, at around 16 weeks, your baby will be roughly the size of an avocado. He or she is a fully formed little person, with a functioning circulatory system and own individual fingerprints!

This can be a transition point in the pregnancy, and it's really important to keep talking to each other, to make sure you both understand how each other feels, so misunderstandings can be avoided.

Pregnancy symptoms can still be present at this point, so discuss together how mum is feeling. What, if anything, is she finding challenging about the pregnancy and is there anything she needs some support with?

When it comes to your relationship with each other, this is a good point to set the habit of talking to each other about how you feel. During pregnancy and after the birth of your baby, as life and feelings quickly change, it can impact on your relationship if you don't communicate.

Pregnancy and parenthood is a period of adjustment for both parents, and you are likely to see some changes to your relationship. Make an effort to be appreciative of each other. Tell your partner that you love him or her, give compliments, thank them for their efforts, whether it is cooking dinner or booking appointments. Be a team.

It either of you believe the myth that all women develop an incredibly high sex drive at a specific point in pregnancy, you might actually start to worry unnecessarily if that doesn't happen! Every couple has their own individual sex lives before pregnancy, and so there is unlikely to be a miraculous change to this just because you are having a baby. If you let go of any expectations of what you think is 'normal' and work instead with what is reality for you as a couple, life can be a lot easier.

If can feel hurtful if your partner does not want to have sex during pregnancy, but it is important to put it in context, and remember all the big life changes going on. There are lots of ways of showing love for each other, so communicate and agree to explore other ways of being intimate until it feels right to resume your sex life. Plan nights out, snuggle together on the sofa watching a movie, go out for lunch, and take a walk together. Thoughtful acts go a long way too – picking up your partner's favourite biscuits, getting him or her a little present 'just because' and so on. It's always nice to be thought of, and this is another real relationship strengthener.

Make time for simple cuddles and affection – this is just as important as sex for keeping your relationship strong, staying connected and showing each other that your deeper feelings have not changed.

CHAPTER 7

Month Five

This month you will reach the halfway point (or thereabouts) in your pregnancy! You will have the opportunity for more medical screenings to check all is well with baby, and may even begin to feel baby moving. There is a lot happening now, and this is often the time from when parents really start to begin their practical preparations for baby!

Hers

Pregnancy symptoms

By this stage, the nausea of morning sickness has usually passed. If you are still struggling with sickness talk to your midwife or doctor for support, and to rule out hyperemesis gravidarum (severe vomiting), which is different from morning sickness.

Noticing aches or discomfort in your lower abdomen or pelvis this month is not uncommon; this is often due to changes in the ligaments and muscles around your pelvis and uterus. During pregnancy your body produces a hormone called relaxin which helps to soften the ligaments and muscles, so that your pelvis can widen ready for birth. A bit of discomfort at this stage is not unusual, but if pelvic pain becomes constant or strong, then talk to your midwife.

You may start to notice symptoms like heartburn, indigestion or constipation. This is also due to the relaxin. As well as softening the pelvic and uterine muscles, relaxin also affects the intestinal muscles which keeps food in your digestive system longer, so you and your baby can absorb more nutrients. Relaxin also relaxes the muscular valve that separates the oesophagus from the stomach, allowing gastric acids to leak upwards.

Due to the increased blood volume in your body during pregnancy, you may experience bleeding gums or nosebleeds.

How do you feel?

As the second antenatal scan comes closer, carried out between 18 – 22 weeks, you may notice a similar mix of feelings from just before the dating scan. Feelings of excitement about seeing your baby on the screen, feelings of worry about potentially finding any problems.

The anomaly scan checks for structural abnormalities (anomalies) in the baby and looks in detail at your baby's bones, heart, brain, spinal cord, face, kidneys and abdomen. It allows the sonographer to look specifically for 11 conditions, some of which are very rare.

The sonographer will also look at what is around baby – the amount of amniotic fluid, the cord flow and where the placenta is positioned.

At this scan the sonographer might identify if the placenta is low-lying, towards the bottom of the uterus. This in itself is only a problem if the placenta is covering the cervix, which baby needs to pass through at the time of birth. However, the majority of placentas move away from the cervix as the pregnancy progresses and the uterus grows, and if you have a low-lying placenta you will be offered the opportunity for another scan at around 32 weeks to recheck its positioning and look at options from there.

His

Your emotions may start to catch up with your partner's at this point in the pregnancy, as her bump begins to show and you see your baby on another scan. You might feel a mix of emotions including excitement and anxiety. As the physical changes become more noticeable in your partner, you may find yourself more concerned about the health and wellbeing of her and your baby. This is often the point where concerns about finances, changes in your relationship and lifestyle and parenting can come to the forefront.

These feelings and thoughts are totally normal, but it is still important to work through any concerns, rather than ignore them. Concerns that we ignore and push away can grow in our subconscious, and can become a bigger problem later on. Going to antenatal classes may address some of the specific concerns you have and you also get to hear from other men in the same boat as you. Check out the useful resources section (see page 223) for more information about antenatal classes.

Your partner

As the second trimester progresses, your partner's physical shape will begin to change to accommodate the growing baby. While a lot of the pregnancy symptoms in the first trimester were related to hormonal changes in pregnancy, in the second trimester, mum also now has other physical changes to contend with on top of this.

The anomaly scan

You will have the opportunity to go for an anomaly scan at around 20 weeks. The primary focus of this scan to is to check your baby's anatomy, and make sure he or she are developing normally. Again, this is a great opportunity to bond with your baby, and if you have been to the first scan already, you will be amazed at how much the baby has developed since then. You may even see your baby wriggling around and kicking!

Get Together

Some exciting things happen this month in the pregnancy – including that your baby starts to be able to see and to hear. What he or she can hear at this stage is mostly the internal sounds of mum's heartbeat or the vibrations of her voice. It will be a little while longer before your baby can hear the outside world. There isn't much to see in the uterus, but your baby will start to be able to recognise the difference between light and dark.

At the end of this month you have the opportunity to attend an anomaly scan. This is a medical screening test, and is offered to look for any potential medical problems with baby or the pregnancy.

A boy or a girl?

Some hospitals offer the opportunity to find out whether your baby is a boy or a girl. However, this is not the point of the test, so whether your hospital will tell you depends on their individual policy. If their policy is not to tell you, you can either wait for a surprise, or pay for a private scan to find out.

If your hospital do disclose the sex on request, then you have a choice! Choosing whether to find out or not can be a tricky decision to make, and of course, everyone has an opinion on whether you should find out or not. Here are some of the things to think about and discuss together before you choose:

■ **Surprise surprise!** Often people say, 'it is nice to have a surprise', and not finding out the sex of your baby until the

birth itself gives you another 20 weeks of letting the anticipation build! However, whenever you choose to find out the
sex of your baby, be it at the 20-week scan, or at the birth,
you always get that wonderful surprise moment! So go with
what feels the best choice for you.

■ **Sexing isn't the point of the scan.** There is an opinion that
parents-to-be focus so much on finding out the gender
that they forget the real reasons behind the ultrasound
scan. It is really important to be mindful that the reason
the scan is being offered is to check on the wellbeing of
your baby and the pregnancy; this is an anomaly scan not
a gender scan. However, it is of course possible to understand this but still plan to find out the sex of your baby.

■ **Mistakes happen!** It is not always possible to get a clear
view of a baby's genitals, to be able to say whether it is a boy
or a girl. Even if the sonographer thinks they can see, there
is also still the possibility of misinterpretation, and they
will warn you it is not a guarantee. Before making your
choice about finding out, it can be worth bearing in mind
how you might feel if you spend half a pregnancy expecting
a baby of one sex and then you get a baby of another! For
some parents, this could be very hard, as they have built a
bond with a baby who they think is a boy/girl and then they
don't get the baby they have been visualising. Other parents
feel they would take it as one of life's great surprises and
have a chuckle about repainting the nursery and sharing
the unexpected news. Consider how do you think you
would feel and does this affect your choice?

■ **A unique kind of birthing incentive?** Whether you choose
to find out or not, you can make it part of your birthing
experience. Not knowing the sex of your baby can be a
real encouragement and help through labour and birth,
knowing you will soon find out. Conversely, knowing the

sex of your baby can give a sense of focus, as you work towards meeting the person you have been picturing for so long.

'In our first birth, we knew the sex and had already chosen the name, so it was incredibly powerful to hear the midwife saying: "In just a couple more contractions you will be meeting Oren." In our fourth birth, we didn't know the sex and it was very powerful knowing we would very soon be discovering whether we had a little boy or girl. No one way was better than the other; they were just different. Whichever choice you make though, it can be used as part of your individual approach to birth.' – **Steph & Dean**

case study

- **Discovering it for yourself.** At a scan someone will tell you whether it is likely your baby is a boy or a girl; it is information that someone else knows first and then gives to you about your baby. If you choose to find out the sex at birth, you can specify on your birth plan that you wish to discover the sex of your baby yourself. This simply means the midwife won't announce: 'It's a boy!' or 'It's a girl!', and you can discover for yourselves. Some couples decide to allow the dad to have the first look and then make the announcement, which gives him a special and memorable role in those moments after baby has arrived.

- **Feeling disappointment.** Plenty of people have experienced a preference for one sex over another, for a variety of reasons. For some, they feel finding out at a scan will enable them to come to terms with any potential disappointment long before the birth and build a bond with their baby. For others, they feel that finding out at the moment of birth when they have their lovely baby in their arms will mean that any disappointment won't be an issue. There is no rule to this, and different things work for different people. Ultimately, it can be normal to have pangs of disappointment whether you find out at a scan or at birth, but rest assured these feelings will pass, and they do not make you a bad parent.

■ **Prevent shopping madness.** Something which you soon discover when you start shopping for baby clothing, is that it can be stereotypically gendered, with lots of pink clothes for girls and blue for boys. If you dislike the idea of gendered clothing, then a way to limit how much might appear in your home would be not finding out the sex. It encourages you and your family shop around for unisex clothing, whether plain white or more colourful. If you are worried you (or another family member) might go overboard on buying things if they know the sex, then not finding out prevents this.

■ **Bonding with the bump.** Knowing the sex of your baby can make it easier to imagine him or her as a little person and start building a bond. You could start choosing a name, as you know it is a name for *them*, not a hypothetical name you may never need. Not knowing the sex of baby can make these things more difficult for some people. If you are having difficulty bonding with your baby in pregnancy, this might be one way of supporting you to develop that bond. Of course, it is also worth remembering that sexing at the scan is not always correct.

■ **Minimising insensitive comments.** If you don't find out the sex of your baby, it can help minimise some of the insensitive and unwelcome comments you might get from friends, family and even strangers. Some people cannot help themselves make comments about the sex, especially if the same sex as your first. Some people will still make such comments after a baby has arrived, but on the whole people tend to be better behaved once baby is here!

The choice to find out or not is yours. It can be useful to decide in advance of the scan, as the moment you are asked: 'Would you like to find out the sex' is not necessarily a decision to make on a whim. It is very tempting to change your mind when asked that question, and, it is, of course, perfectly fine to change your mind, but chatting it through together first will enable you to make a decision that you both feel happy with.

If you do find out the sex, you do not have to tell the world if you don't wish to. You could find out and keep it a secret between yourselves.

CHAPTER 8

Month Six

Every pregnancy is different, but this month is often the one where your baby has grown enough to start to be more visibly noticeable as a 'bump', and dad may now be able to feel baby kicking when his hand is placed on mum's abdomen. It's also time to start to make plans about working arrangements following this birth, so as usual, there are a few things to plan and discuss!

Hers

Pregnancy symptoms

This month, your growing bump changes your centre of gravity, so it is not unusual to feel a little unsteady now and again. Your uterus is higher than your belly button at this point in the pregnancy, which means the skin around your abdomen and breasts will be stretching to accommodate it, and might feel dry or itchy.

You may be experiencing nasal congestion and find yourself snoring for the first time in your life! This is due to the swelling of the mucous membranes.

Your blood pressure can fall during pregnancy, a result of all the extra blood your body has to pump around; this can leave you feeling lightheaded as you stand up from sitting, or feeling faint if you have to be on your feet a long time. Learn what your body can do, and if you need a rest, take one.

'Being on my feet for any length of time is just very difficult – I always end up feeling faint, and once I did faint in a shop! Now, if I have to go out, I make sure that I can sit down (even if that means being the pregnant women who sits on the floor in a queue!) or where possible, I order online and have shopping delivered.' – **Pam**

case study

Planning maternity leave

If you are in employment, it is helpful to start thinking about maternity leave this month, if you have not done so already. You need to let your employer know when you intend your leave to begin, about 15 weeks before your baby is due (week 25 of your pregnancy). In the UK, pregnant women are entitled to 52 weeks of maternity leave, no matter how long they've worked for their employer. This is made up of 26 weeks of 'ordinary' maternity leave and 26 weeks of 'additional' maternity leave. How much you get paid during this year will depend on your contract, so this is a good time to check if you don't know. There is a statutory minimum.

Deciding when you wish to begin your maternity leave can be a difficult decision. Some women want to have as much time as possible with their baby, so opt to take maternity leave as close to the birth as possible. Other women decide that they want some time to prepare and rest before baby arrives, especially if commuting or working while pregnant is challenging.

It is pretty common to have mixed feelings about planning leave, especially if you enjoy your work and get on well with your colleagues. Sometimes we can feel guilty about taking time away, but try not to worry about letting people down; your workplace will manage without you! When you decide to start your leave can be influenced by a range of factors:

- How long is your commute?
- Can you work from home some of the time?
- How challenging/tiring is your work?
- How are you finding your pregnancy?
- How much are you enjoying working?
- Do you need/want to prioritise leave for after the birth?
- Do you plan to return to work, and if so, at what time?

It is helpful to remember that pregnancy reaches full term at 37 weeks – which means if you went into labour at this point, it would be normal, not early. It is not unheard of for women to stop working at 37 weeks and give birth the next day! When you think about how the body works (see page 129) this makes sense – as maternity leave begins, you feel a sense of relief and relaxation, which enables the flow of oxytocin, and so thus starts labour!

Conversely, normal term can also continue up to 42 weeks of pregnancy, so it is also worth considering how you will feel if this is the case for you. If you decide to start maternity leave several weeks before baby arrives, will the waiting make you feel more impatient and stressed?

There is no right or wrong when it comes to deciding when you want maternity leave to begin, and it doesn't matter what work colleagues or friends or family have done or expect. Decide what feels right for you based on how you're feeling. If you want to start your leave at 29 weeks, you can do so. If you want to work up until 40 weeks, you can do that too. What feels right for your own situation, your body and your baby?

As well as working out when you want your maternity leave to begin, you may also be giving thought to when it will end. Some women prefer to take a year off work and see how things go, and how they feel once baby has arrived. However, for various reasons, others need to plan to return to work at a set point after the birth.

You may need to start looking into childcare arrangements earlier rather than later, even before your baby is born. It's not always easy to find childcare that suits what you need and that you feel comfortable with, so be aware that it may take you some time.

His

Although it may still feel like a way off, this month is the time to start putting into place arrangements for your paternity leave. In the UK fathers are entitled to at least two weeks' paternity leave following the birth. Depending on your employer, you may be offered longer than this, but this is the minimum you can expect if you wish to take it. How much you get paid will depend on your contract and duration of employment. You will need to let your employer know of your intention to take paternity leave 15 weeks before your baby is due (week 25 of your partner's pregnancy).

Paternity leave is important and has so many benefits for you, your partner and your baby. It gives you crucial bonding time with your baby, as well as time to learn about how to care for him or her, and how to get stuck in with being an active and hands-on dad. The more you are involved, the more confident you will feel, and the more confident in you your partner and baby will also feel.

Paternity leave is also shown to be hugely beneficial in establishing breastfeeding. One study showed that when fathers took paternity leave, their partners and babies were significantly more likely to be still breastfeeding at two, four and six months. Having support and care from their partners in those first few days when learning a new skill, makes a difference to how confident, competent and supported a woman is likely to feel. Support to get breastfeeding off to a good start, and the opportunity for dad to learn how he can support mum, has a long-lasting impact.

It is not uncommon for men to feel a sense of anxiety or pressure when it comes to providing for the family. The desire to look after and protect the economic wellbeing of the nest can mean that we feel we need to get back to work as quickly as possible. While this is undoubtedly important, so is being with your family, and it can be helpful to think about how you can balance the two. Look at options like taking annual leave instead of paternity leave to maintain a salary, or budgeting before baby arrives to allow you to take time off without having to worry about money.

If leave is important to you as a family, it is helpful to make sure your plans are informed. One study looking at fatherhood highlighted the numbers of fathers who said they 'cannot afford' to take paternity leave. Interestingly, in the majority of those cases, it was an assumption, rather than a fact based on financial calculations.

You may feel different when you return to work after the arrival of your baby. Some dads find having to leave their new family behind brings feelings of guilt, jealousy or resentment. You might feel as though you are missing out. Your baby changes and grows so quickly, you might sometimes resent the fact that you are not there to see it all. You might feel jealous that your partner got to see something special, and you missed it. You might feel guilty if something happens and you are not there to be a part of it. Sometimes these feelings can be quite overwhelming, and you can take them out on your partner by being critical or snapping at her. Being aware of your feelings, and why you are feeling them, is the first step in helping prevent this happen. It is a pretty vulnerable time for both of you.

You might notice that you feel different about work after the arrival of your baby. Even dads who love their work can feel they no longer want to stay late in the office, but rather get home to be with their family. This can cause difficulties if colleagues have expectations of you, but your priorities have changed. This happens more often than is discussed, and can possibly be attributed to the fact that men go through hormonal changes too. Studies show that new dads can experience a drop in testosterone levels of up to 30 per cent, which, it is hypothesised, is nature's way of ensuring dad becomes a more stable parent. This can mean that even the most career-minded of men suddenly find that work just isn't that important any more and that family is.

Get Together

B y the end of this month, your baby will look like a perfectly formed little person! The eyebrows and eyelids are fully developed, and he or she has tiny little fingernails. At 24 weeks your pregnancy also reaches a big milestone, as it becomes 'viable' in medical terms. This means that if your baby was born prematurely now, there would be a chance of survival with a lot of specialist medical support.

It is helpful to make time to discuss your options for maternity and paternity leave together well before baby arrives, so you can start to put any practical arrangements into action. You will both need to give your workplaces notice that you intend to take maternity/paternity leave. You may be surprised at the preferences of your partner, and have more options to explore. Key points to discuss might include:

- How long do you wish to have on leave?
- How long would you like your partner to take off?
- What is important to you about your/their leave?

Every person, and every couple is different, and discussing together your vision for those first weeks with your baby will help create a shared understanding and set the pathway to make it possible.

It is also important in making sure that you get to consider all of your options. In the UK you may be eligible to share parental leave and pay. Shared parental leave is designed to give parents the flexibility to decide when to return to work and how to spend time together in the early stages of a child's life. Leave can be taken separately or at the same time.

Be mindful of the things which you both feel you might be missing out on, and work together to overcome those. Some dads arrange to take their baby to a swimming or massage class while mum has a lie-in, so they get some special daddy-and-baby time while their partner has some rest. There are lots of potential options to making the most of time even after leave has come to an end.

CHAPTER 9

Month Seven

As you go into this month you may be noticing how rapidly mum's body is growing and changing, bringing the thought of the birth more to your mind. This is a great time in the pregnancy to start looking into your antenatal preparation options, and to make arrangements to attend classes.

Hers

Pregnancy symptoms

Your uterus has grown up near your ribcage which can mean bouts of breathlessness. If you have breathlessness with notable fatigue and/or palpitations, mention this to your midwife, as it could be that you have pregnancy anaemia. If you attend an antenatal appointment this month, you may be offered a blood test to check your iron levels. As the amount of fluids in your body increases, the red blood cells that contain iron may not adequately keep pace, which can cause lower haemoglobin levels causing pregnancy anaemia. Many pregnant women develop this, and it can be treated by dietary changes or iron supplements.

You may also have started to experience another pregnancy delight – varicose veins. Women are more prone to these during pregnancy, due to the weight of the growing baby and placenta on the large vein (inferior vena cava) which returns blood from the lower limbs to the heart. Also, increased blood volume, along with the pregnancy hormone progesterone relaxing your blood vessel walls, means that varicose veins is not unusual.

Most commonly, women experience varicose veins in their legs, but you can get them in other parts of your body. Haemorrhoids (piles) are basically varicose veins of the rectal area, and are very common in pregnancy. Some women develop varicose veins in and around their vagina. If you have any concerns or discomfort, talk to your midwife. The good news is that in most cases, these will gradually disappear after pregnancy.

How do you feel?

As your bump starts to get bigger and baby's movements get stronger, the idea of birth becomes more real. This is a great time to start your antenatal education preparations and learn more about what to expect and your choices. Remember that what you have seen and heard on TV or from friends is not necessarily representative of how birth is, or indeed, how it will be for you. Just like pregnancy, every birth is different! The topic for the 'get together' at the end of this chapter is about the choices available in antenatal education, so make time to discuss how and what you would like to do to prepare for both the birth of your baby, but also caring for them once they have arrived.

Tuning into your baby

Tuning into our baby's movements is really beneficial in terms of helping us to build that bond with them before they have even arrived. However, more than this, it is also important to do, as our baby's movements are an indicator of how they are coping with life in the uterus.

Every baby is individual and their pattern of movements will be unique to them. Some babies move more or less than others, or have specific times of day when they are very active. Your body position and movements may also encourage movement; some babies move about when you are eating or drinking, or you may notice specific foods (or temperatures of food and drink) cause movement. When you tune into your baby's activity, you can start to notice these kinds of patterns, and learn what is usual for your baby.

Your baby moving in their usual way, is a way of them communicating that all is well. When a baby is poorly or in distress for some reason, there can be a change to their pattern of movements. Guidance from NICE (National Institute for Health and Care Excellence) states that: 'Any changes in foetal movements should be reported to a midwife or healthcare professional for further assessment.'

There is a myth that all babies movements slow down towards the end of pregnancy because they 'run out of space' or are 'conserving their energy for labour'. It is important that you know that this isn't true. As a baby gets bigger they do have less room to move around, and this can make the movements feel different, but how regular they are and the usual timings will remain the same until they are born. Don't assume it is normal for a reduction of movements later in pregnancy, and if you notice any change to what is normal for your baby, talk immediately to a midwife. Don't wait for your next antenatal appointment; call the maternity outpatients clinic at your local hospital – it is why it is there.

You can track baby's movements in a couple of ways: you can buy a 'kick counter' bracelet to keep track of how many movements you feel (see page 224). You could also just choose a quiet time of the day when you tune into your baby, and keep a note of how many movements you feel.

His

This is often the month when you can start to really connect with your unborn baby in a new way, as they can start to hear your voice and you may start to feel their movements!

During this month, by around 24 weeks, your baby can hear sounds from outside. This means that your baby can now hear your voice, and is getting to know you and is bonding with you. You may also feel your baby move or kick for the first time. It can take a bit of patience to feel a kick; you need to keep your hand on the bump for a while and not give up after five minutes, as, inevitably, the moment you take your hand away is when baby will move! This game of hide-and-seek is all part of the fun and is a great opportunity to become physically connected and bonded with your baby.

Why not make time to sit down together with your partner to try and feel your baby moving around. Maybe offer your partner a snack or a massage while you sit together, and make it a lovely experience all round. Showing effort and interest towards your baby and the pregnancy, has benefits for your relationship, as she will feel that you value both her and the baby. Pregnancy, and the early days with a newborn, can be tough on relationships, so building a strong foundation now is so important.

Bonding with your baby is also important for your own confidence. You will find that the more connected you feel during pregnancy, the more comfortable you will feel when your newborn arrives. Your baby will also sense this inner-confidence, and feel more secure and safe with you as a result, which will help keep baby feel calm and bonded with you!

Your baby's movements are also an important part of signalling that all is well with the pregnancy. If your baby starts to move less, or significantly more than usual, this may indicate difficulties. If your partner ever, at any point in the pregnancy, feels that the baby is not moving as usual, support her to be checked at the local hospital right away. You can be the one to call to explain the situation and ask to be seen right away. A midwife will monitor baby's heartbeat and movements, and most of the time all will be well. Occasionally, tests might show that baby is in difficulty, and getting baby checked has led to lives being saved.

All of this bonding with baby can make the upcoming birth appear all the more immediate and real. As your partner continues to grow and baby's movements become stronger over the next weeks, the reality of birth starts to loom for her too. So if you haven't already, this is also a good time to start planning your antenatal education.

The majority of fathers in the UK attend antenatal classes. This is a great way to learn what to expect during labour and birth, how to support your partner, and to learn about life with a newborn baby.

If you plan on being the birth partner, you need to prepare. Research shows that birth partners affect the length of labour, the degree of pain your partner may or may not feel, and whether interventions such as caesarean sections are required. Your role at the birth matters and can really make a difference. Antenatal classes are your opportunity to make sure you are doing everything you can to ensure that your presence at the birth is a positive one. It is definitely not all up to your partner to learn on her own! This is your opportunity to get involved in preparing for birth and fatherhood, and to work out what path you want to take together.

Get Together

T his month your baby's brain is going through some crucial development, but he or she are also undergoing many physical changes. The buds for their baby teeth have already formed in the gums, and your baby may also start to open and blink their eyes! Your baby has grown large enough now that it might be possible to feel them hiccupping; this may feel like small kicks, but will have a rhythmical pattern to them.

As you enter into the second half of pregnancy, it is a good time to start thinking about what kind of birth preparations you would both like to do. There are now a wide range of antenatal classes available to help you prepare for the kind of birth you would like to have.

Discuss together what you would like your birth to be like. Try to focus on the positives of how you would like your birth to be, rather than anything negative you have heard about or seen. You can then research what classes are available in your area, and make sure you attend the ones that suit how you feel about your birth. For example, if you are hoping to have a birth without using drugs, then it makes sense to attend a class which specifically teaches natural coping techniques and skills, rather than a hospital-based class focusing on using medical pain relief.

'When I was pregnant with our first baby, I really didn't want an epidural. It was only in the middle of labour when I was struggling with the contractions that I realised I hadn't learnt anything at our antenatal classes to help me cope! Our classes had focused on the choices of pain relief available, which given I didn't want to use them, wasn't helpful for me.

For our second and subsequent births, I made sure that I learnt skills to help me with my preference of not using medical pain relief, and had a more positive experience as a result!' – **Anne**

case study

There is no rule saying you can attend only one kind of class; some parents do a few so they have different resources, information and techniques to hand.

It might be that you attend some classes together, or that one or both of you also go to some separately – it doesn't matter, just whatever suits you both and what you each want to learn.

What are the options?

Gone are the days when there were only very basic antenatal preparation classes on offer; there is now a wide choice, meaning that you can choose something that will provide what you want to get from them.

There may be free classes run by the NHS in your area, and your midwife can tell you about them. These vary widely in terms of how they are run and the content.

There are many private classes available too; find out what is on offer in your local area which appeal to what and how you want to learn about birth and parenting. Choose a class or classes which are accredited (so you know they are being well run).

Classes that cover coping strategies for birth will include breathing practice, relaxation, ways of working with the body to make birthing easier and ways of feeling more confident about giving birth. There is often the choice of doing these classes in female-only groups, or together as a couple.

Growing in popularity are male-only classes for expectant dads, and of course we were pioneers in developing DaddyNatal – classes for men facilitated by male antenatal facilitators to really enhance the experience. These focus on the specific skills and information dads-to-be need to know in their role as birth partner. They also give men the opportunity to meet others going through the same life changes, and to be able to be open and frank about their experiences.

Classes that include teaching skills for caring for your newborn are also invaluable. From deciding how and if you would like vitamin K administered to your baby after birth (see page 208), to learning how to bathe your baby – specific classes allowing you to get understanding and hands-on with all of these options are very helpful.

Some hospitals offer tours of the birthing wards, either through visits, or virtual online tours. Look out too for Home Birth information days, run by the NHS, which are really helpful if giving birth at home is a choice you would like more information about.

Some hospitals and clinics offer breastfeeding workshops. While breastfeeding might seem like something that doesn't have a lot to do with dads, studies show that dads have a huge impact on mum's breastfeeding relationship, so if breastfeeding is something you and your partner have decided you would like to do, attending these classes can be very useful to help you achieve your aim.

For some links to good antenatal providers, look at the further information and resources section at the back of the book (see page 223).

When should we attend?

Most classes suggest you start in the third trimester of pregnancy (from 27 weeks) so that all the participants' babies are due around the same time. However, it is up to you when you want to attend, if you prefer to go earlier or later. Some classes run over several weeks so make sure you can fit it all in before reaching full term at 37 weeks!

Can dads take time off work to attend?

Since October 2014 in the UK, dads-to-be have the right to take unpaid time off work to accompany their partners for up to two antenatal appointments, which include antenatal classes. If you have already used your time off to attend other appointments, you can still request time off to attend, or take annual leave.

Antenatal classes are run over a wide variety of week-days, evenings and weekends though – so if you can't attend the first ones you find, keep looking around for something else which will suit your individual circumstances. Some antenatal providers will even come to your home and run classes for you at a time which does suit you both. There might be classes close to your work which fit in better, al-though this does mean that the parents you meet may not live near you.

What do you want to get out of antenatal classes?

Whatever antenatal class you choose, you should leave feel-ing prepared for birth and the early days of parenting. This means feeling confident that you understand how the body works in labour and birth, how to work with it, that you un-derstand your choices, and that you feel supported to explore what feels right to you as a family.

Try talking to a couple of providers about what approach and information their classes focus on. Ask other people who have attended classes how they felt their classes prepared them and impacted on their birth experience. While it is nice to attend antenatal classes to make friends (as developing a peer network is really beneficial), this is just one aspect of what antenatal classes should aim to achieve, so this is worth keeping in mind.

Not all antenatal classes are equal or suitable for everyone, so if you attend a class and you don't feel that you are learning what you need to know, or it is not making you feel more confident about what is to come, try another one while you have time. Like many things in life, different things suit different people and it is important to make sure that you find the right fit for your family.

CHAPTER 10

Month Eight

By the end of this month, your pregnancy will be almost 'full term' meaning that meeting your baby may not be far away. Being heavily pregnant can be tough, so take things steadily and begin those final preparations to make sure you are ready for the arrival of your little one!

Hers

Pregnancy symptoms

At this point in the pregnancy, you may start to notice swelling around your fingers, ankles, feet and/or face. Swelling is extremely common in pregnancy; it is thought to affect nearly half of all pregnant women. Swelling will often become more apparent in hands or feet as the day goes on because the fluids that cause swelling are affected by gravity, and drain down to the feet and hands.

If you find yourself dealing with this symptom, there are a few things you can do. These may not get rid of all the swelling, but they can help minimise it and improve your comfort:

- Drink lots of water to help your kidneys filter the excess fluids.
- Rest as much as you can with your feet elevated.
- If you need to stand for any length of time, try shifting your weight from foot to foot, so each leg is rested in turn.
- Circle your feet or hands one way, then the other.
- At night time, pop a pillow under your feet, so that gravity can drain the fluids away from the feet and ankles.
- If you find your shoes do not fit, you may need to go shopping for new, more comfortable ones. If pregnant in summer, many women wear flip flops to prevent their feet having to be squeezed into shoes.

Most swelling in pregnancy is normal, however if you notice swelling which comes on very suddenly, is severe, or if you just are not sure, contact your midwife right away. Severe or rapid onset of swelling can be a symptom of other medical conditions like Pre-eclampsia, which may need attention.

Preparing the birth bags.

Getting your birth bags ready is an exciting and sometimes daunting part of pregnancy, as it signals that things are getting close at hand! You may feel excited as you get ready, or have flutters of nervousness. You are likely to feel both these things from time to time.

As birth will usually occur anytime from 37 weeks, it is a good idea to get the birth bags prepared before this point of your pregnancy, so that you can ease some of those nerves, knowing that you are ready for whenever it may be.

Whether you are choosing to have your baby at home or at hospital, it is a handy to have some bags with the essentials in, as this keeps them all organised and to hand. Of course, not everything you may want to use will fit in a bag – you may wish to have a birth ball or a pillow to use too.

What should I pack?

Birth bags, like birth plans, vary from person to person. Everyone has a different view of what they need to feel comfortable during birth and in the hours afterwards.

There are a few key things which are usually helpful, and this list will help you get started:

- Your birth plan.
- Any medication you are taking.
- A nightie or big T-shirt for labour. If you are planning to use a bath or birthing pool take a bikini top so you have the option to cover up if you like.
- Energy-giving snacks for labour such as dried fruits and flapjacks. Take a bottle of squash or similar for a refreshing and energising drink.
- Anything else you feel will help to make your birth environment cosy and comfortable, such as a pillow, birth ball, photos of loved ones, music, a favourite cuddly toy. We call these birth anchors, and they are especially important if you are birthing away from home, as the smell, feel and appearance can bring us comfort and security.
- Front-opening nightwear and breastfeeding bras if choosing to breastfeed.
- Toothbrush, toothpaste, tissues, flannel, towel, shampoo, body wash and hairbands for long hair. Small travel-size bottles can help with space.
- Dressing gown, slippers and anything else that feels comfortable and useful for after the birth.
- Sanitary towels for after the birth. Look for specific postnatal pads which are designed for heavier blood loss. You can use standard disposable pads which are available in most supermarkets, or look to purchase reusable cloth pads which require washing but can be more comfortable. Tampons are not advised due to the high risk of infection following birth.

- Plenty of loose fitting knickers. Whatever kind of pads you use, you are likely to have leaks from time to time, and so have lots of pairs. You could use disposable knickers or buy some cheap cotton knickers.
- If birthing in hospital, clothes for coming home. Choose something that is loose and comfortable, and bear in mind that it is unlikely that you will fit into pre-maternity clothes straight away.

His

As the reality of birth and parenthood looms even closer this month, it is time to start making those essential preparations, if you haven't already!

For dads who are planning to be birth partner, an important part of your role is looking after the 'birth bags' – making sure they are packed into the car and taken with you to hospital, or on hand as required at home if birthing there.

Even if your partner takes the lead on organising the stuff you need, you still need to get involved. Find out what is in each bag and also where it is in the bag. If your partner needs something in the middle of labour, or quickly after the birth of your baby, you need to be able to find it.

It is useful to have your own birth bag, which contains things you might need as birth partner, and to take care of yourself. As it would be completely normal for labour to begin anytime from week 37, make sure you have your stuff ready before this. How prepared you are in packing your bag can send signals to your partner about how seriously you are taking your role, and can help her feel relaxed. Make this a task which you take care of without needing prompts or reminders, and let her know, without expecting praise, when you have done it.

What should I pack?

- Birth plan. You can't have enough copies of this, so make sure you pack a copy too.
- Make sure you have supply of food and drink for yourself. Glucose energy drinks are great, although be mindful if they have added caffeine or other stimulants, how much you are consuming. Add some cereal bars, nuts or crisps that can stay in the bag until needed. Make some sandwiches when early labour begins and pop them into your bag too, for both you and your partner. You do not want to be passing out at a crucial moment in the birth because you have not eaten for hours, nor do you want to be the dad who misses the birth because he was in the café!
- An easy drinking bottle or a couple of bendy straws. Keeping your partner hydrated in labour is extremely important, as dehydration can slow down labour and make it painful. Something she can sip from easily, in any position, will help a lot.
- A flannel. You can use this as a warm compress (run under a warm tap) on the lower back during labour to offer relief. As labour really gets underway, and your partner is getting hot and sweaty, wet the flannel under a cold tap to use as a cold compress on her face; this can give relief and revitalise.
- Your phone, so you can share the news or get that first photo.

Get Together

B y the end of this month, your baby has fully grown fingernails and toenails. The central nervous system is still maturing, but the lungs are nearly fully developed. If either of you have been anxious about the possibility of your baby being born prematurely, *the good news is that 99 per cent of babies born at this point will have no major health problems.*

As you get nearer to 37 weeks, having your birth bags ready is a good idea. As there are a few things you might need, it can be handy to have three bags: one for mum, one for dad and one for the baby. Decide who is going to get the baby things ready, and what you need.

If you both pack your own bags, then that can leave the things to pack for your baby. If you are birthing at home, you also have some things you need to get ready too, so it can be helpful to discuss who is going to do what.

Birth bag for baby

- Cord tie for your baby's cord, if you are opting to use (see page 206).
- Baby vests and baby grows – if birthing at home having a couple of these to hand is useful, if going into hospital take a few more in case you stay in a couple of days. Newborn sizes will fit most babies, even if for a short time.
- Baby blanket. Hospitals will have plenty, but you might like to take your own too. You can use the blanket for when baby naps, when you are holding him or her, and for the journey home.
- A pack of nappies. You can choose disposables, reusable or hybrids (which have a reusable outer wrap, but a disposable inner lining). Whichever type you want to use is up to you, and all are suitable from birth.
- Cotton wool or cloth wipes and a plastic bowl for nappy changing. Advice is to just use water to clean baby's bottom for the first few weeks, so using cotton wool or cloth wipes is an easy way of doing this.
- Muslin cloths. These are to protect your clothes when you are holding baby, as some babies will posset a little milk after feeding.

- A special 'coming home' piece of clothing to wear for baby. You don't need this, but if you have found something special, why not take it along. Some parents then choose to keep the outfit for a memory box.
- A snowsuit or jacket if the weather is cold – although be aware not to use padded jackets or snowsuits in car seats, as they do not allow the harness to be properly fitted, meaning baby is not properly restrained in the event of an accident.
- A car seat is essential for taking baby home in the car. Practice how it fits into the car, and work out how the straps fit together before you try it with your baby inside!

Getting ready for a home birth

If you are giving birth at home there will be a few additional things that you need to have at the ready. These include:

- A birth pool, if you have chosen to use one. You can hire or purchase a pool.
- Waterproof sheet – to protect the floor or furniture during birthing and immediately afterwards.
- Towels.
- A torch.
- Warm water and antibacterial soap.

More information about home birth can be found in later in the book (see page 124).

And finally

Each couple is different in terms of their birth plan and needs, so it's important to talk to each other about what you want and need and make sure you pack accordingly!

You want to strike a balance between packing the things you will want and need, and packing several suitcases worth! Remember that you can always pop home (if in hospital) or to the shop after baby has been born if you find there is something you do need which you haven't got yet.

CHAPTER 11

Month Nine and beyond

This month, at 37 weeks of pregnancy, you become 'full term', meaning it is perfectly normal for your baby to be born and there is no medical need to try and stop labour if it begins. Not all babies arrive by the 'estimated due date' which will be at the end of this month, as it is perfectly normal for a baby to arrive any time up until 42 weeks, and some babies may arrive a little later than this too.

Hers

Pregnancy symptoms

You may find this stage of pregnancy can be physically tough. You may experience heartburn, constipation, wind, piles, cramps and dizziness. As the skin on your stomach continues to stretch, you may have very itchy skin. You may be getting tired, and need to rest or nap more. As your uterus pushes up against the bottom of your ribcage, you may have discomfort and breathlessness. Your belly button may be stretched and start to protrude – this is perfectly normal and is not permanent. Your baby will be putting more pressure on your bladder, meaning you need frequent toilet stops and wake up in the night more often.

Despite feeling like this, you may also experience the famous 'nesting' instinct, and feel an urge to clean your home from top to bottom, and finish off any jobs that need doing!

How do you feel?

You may feel a sense of anticipation as you get closer to your due date, but then find that it flies by and you are still pregnant. You might feel frustrated even if you knew it was likely to happen. Try and take things one day at a time, rather than thinking, 'I might still be pregnant in a week!' Labour can begin quickly, and there is no saying that even if you start the day pregnant and with no signs, that you won't end the day with your baby in your arms.

When you find yourself feeling impatient or frustrated, try to remind yourself that you are not overdue at 40 weeks. You are not 'post-term' until you are 42 weeks, and even then you still have the choice to wait for your body to go into labour naturally. Remember that your due date is an estimate, not a deadline. Practical ideas for staying positive during these last few weeks include:

- **Rest.** Things always feel worse the more tired you are. Rest as much as you can during the day, and take naps whenever you feel like them, especially if you are struggling to sleep properly at night.

- **Use the time productively.** Do things now to make those first days easier when your baby arrives, such as cooking and freezing meals that you will be able to heat up after baby arrives.

- **Try relaxation and meditation.** If you have learnt these skills to use during your birth, you could practise now for when needed during labour and birth, and to help you to feel calmer during pregnancy. You may find that they also help you rest and sleep better too.

- **Try some gentle exercise.** Go for a swim or a gentle walk. Exercise boosts endorphins and mood.

- **Celebrate still being pregnant.** This might sound strange, but if you are going to still be pregnant at this point, why not make the most of it? You could get some photos of you, make a belly cast with some help from your partner, or even paint your bump!

His

This last month can be tough on your partner. Physically, being heavily pregnant can be hard work and very tiring. Your partner may be finding it tough to sleep due to frequent trips to the toilet, practise contractions (see page 130), or just difficulty getting comfortable in bed. Add in heartburn, swelling, pelvic pain, haemorrhoids or other symptoms ... one of these on their own can be tough, but when all put together, it is something else!

On top of this, her emotions may start to become very strong. Physical discomforts can make anyone feel irritable, and being the person closest to her, you might have this taken out on you. Try to not take it to heart; it can be a difficult point in the pregnancy for some women.

Your partner may start to feel anxious about labour and birth as the realisation dawns that it really could be any day now. She may find herself feeling impatient and fed up, not helped by people constantly asking her: 'Haven't you had that baby yet?' and calling to see if there is news.

If you notice that your partner is feeling anxious about giving birth, or she tells you so, the most important thing is not to dismiss how she feels, or just say: 'It'll be fine', or something similar. Not making a big deal of it might be helpful in avoiding to feed a fear, but enabling her to say how she feels, and listening to her, can be an important part of the process of her dealing with any fears she has. You don't have to solve them, but you can reassure her that the vast majority of mums and babies are fine.

You can support her by spending time doing positive preparations, rather than on worrying about things which only 'might' happen. If you have done antenatal classes, either together or separately, practise the skills and tools you have learnt. If she has done some classes or learnt some skills on her own, ask her to show you what she has learnt, so that she can feel more calm and confident that you understand what she wants to use to cope during birth and can support her to do so.

Show her that you are taking your role as the birth partner seriously. If you are confident and prepared, that will help ease her anxiety. You might choose to stop drinking alcohol (in case you need to be 'on duty' for the birth), work closer to home if you can, read this book, make sure all the birth bags are ready, double-check the birth plan, and offer to go with her to any antenatal appointments. Moral support at this point in the pregnancy can go a long way.

Get Together

Once you have reached the end of week 36, your baby is considered 'full term', which means it would be perfectly normal for your baby to be born any day now. Each baby develops at *his or her own pace, so the challenge this month is staying patient until they are ready to make an appearance.*

Although you have an estimated due date (EDD), it is impossible to know exactly when your baby will arrive. Even if you have a scheduled caesarean booked in the diary, there is no saying that will definitely be the day baby arrives, as it is possible baby might try to arrive earlier – which would mean their birth would be brought forward.

You will have an estimated due date (EDD), which is either determined by a set of measurements of your baby at the Dating Scan if you choose to have one, or by the date of mum's last period. Your EDD is really just one date in the middle of an entire five-week window of when would be normal for your baby to be born (any time between 37–42 weeks of pregnancy). Knowing this gives you more choice when it comes to choosing induction or not, (see page 115), and can also help with coping with those last weeks of pregnancy.

Understanding this 'window' means that your baby is not 'early' if born between 37–40 weeks, and not 'late' if born between 40–42 weeks. Babies who are born any time in that 5 week window are still on time! It's important to know, because less than 5 per cent of babies are actually born on their EDD, which can lead to parents being shocked and unprepared if their baby arrives much earlier than this, or feeling impatient and as though their body isn't doing what it should, if their baby is later than this. The reality is, that anywhere between 37–42 weeks in perfectly normal and on time!

With this in mind, it is helpful to not focus too much on a single date, but to be prepared for how it is perfectly normal for the birth to be any time in those few weeks. The due date is a guide, not a deadline!

Many families are now even choosing to not tell other people their due dates, so that they are not inundated with phone calls and messages in the weeks and days in the lead up asking for baby news! Being under the microscope in this way can make everything feel as though it is taking so much longer and make you feel under increased pressure. Instead of saying they are due on the 17th March, for example, many parents are now choosing to say 'we are due in March'.

Your baby may not have arrived by the EDD because he or she is simply not ready. Each baby develops in the uterus at their own pace, and some are ready before others. In those last few weeks, your baby is still doing some critical growth; crucially the lungs are undergoing final development, to be able to breathe air after birth.

However, even understanding this, we are all human and those last weeks can be hard. It is always a nice idea to plan a celebration for your due date, so that if you are still pregnant that day (and it is very possible that you will be!) that you have a positive focus for the day. Plan to go out for a meal or something nice. In fact, a little treat a day in those last few weeks of waiting can be a good plan! The more relaxed and at ease mum feels, the more likely her labour will begin. The more stressed you are, the more likely you are going to be producing hormones which inhibit labour starting. If you ever need an excuse for some daily pampering, this is it!

As you reach 40 weeks of pregnancy, you are likely to be offered a 'stretch and sweep', which is a form of induction (see page 196). It is always a choice to accept or decline any induction offered, so discuss together the pros and cons, and how having this intervention fits in with your birth plan. This can be a good point in your pregnancy to revisit your birth plan, and remember that choices made before labour begins can impact on the course of labour and birth itself.

If friends and family ringing or messaging you every day to find out how things are going is frustrating you, ask them to stop! Many women and their partners post a message or image on social media accounts saying: 'We'll tell you when we've had the baby!' (or similar), to give people the hint not to keep asking. Discuss together how you want to handle any over-enthusiastic friends and family.

section three

Labour and Birth

CHAPTER 12

Birth preferences

One thing you are likely to hear when you are pregnant is the phrase, 'there is no point having a birth plan'. This simply isn't true. Is it true that not all births go according to plan? Of course. But then, in life we plan a variety of things which also don't always go exactly how we have envisaged them – that is the nature of the unpredictability of life! However, it doesn't stop us having a plan ... We plan weddings, parties, holidays, meals, travel ... the list is endless. Sometimes things go awry or there is something unexpected we haven't accounted for, and we have to adapt a plan, but for the most part, we all plan all the time.

Hers

It is useful to think of the birth plan, not as a 'wish list', but rather as your view on the approach and preferences you have around your birth. One of the biggest benefits of writing a birth plan is that it can give you both the opportunity to research and understand all the different options and choices available.

From where you would prefer your baby to be born, to whether and for how long you would like delayed cord clamping after the birth – a birth plan isn't just about pain relief or type of birth.

Sometimes aspects of a birth plan are only more likely to be fulfilled if you take actions before your birth itself. Decisions we make during pregnancy can impact our birth experience, and therefore being aware of these can dramatically change how likely our plan is to be fulfilled.

For example, if your preference is to give birth without using drugs, then it can be helpful to think about what you DO want to do to support you to achieve this in labour. This is all part of your birth planning – this might mean doing antenatal classes which teach you specific skills to use in labour and then during your pregnancy, practising those skills. Then instead of your birth plan saying 'I don't want an epidural' you could choose to write 'I will be using mindful breathing and relaxation practices to cope with labour, so please support me and remind me to use these.' This then signals to the midwife, not just what you don't want, but how you actually want them to support you. While this doesn't guarantee your preference, it makes it more likely to happen.

Another example might be, if your preference is for no interventions and a straightforward vaginal birth, understanding that consenting to an intervention before labour has begun (such as induction) will reduce the likelihood of that birth plan preference. This doesn't mean you should or shouldn't have an induction (every situation is different) but understanding that a choice you make before labour has started is likely to impact on how it goes, is very important. Understanding that, you can then choose whether to consent to an induction, consent to aspects of an induction, delay an induction, decline an induction. It also enables you to understand that practices like a stretch and sweep are also an intervention and can impact on birth plans. We look in more detail at the topic of induction in Chapter 19, but given it has such a large bearing on birth, and now 1 in 4 births are induced, it is a consideration which should be part of everybody's birth planning.

Something we have heard a lot over the years is parents-to-be saying, 'I'll go with the flow'. I find this interesting and always ask – 'whose flow?' The flow of your own body and baby during labour? The flow of the medical environment? The flow of the preferences of the specific midwife you have looking after you by chance? The reality is that these are likely to all be different 'flows'. The flow of midwives looking after you at a home birth is likely to be quite different to the 'flow' of midwives looking after you on a busy delivery suite in a hospital, for example. A midwife who is more comfortable with supporting women to have active births, might have a different flow to a midwife who is more comfortable with supporting women who have epidurals. None of these are right or wrong, but 'going with the flow' suggests you have no preferences as to what happens, and usually this isn't the case. Even if you think you are going with the flow, you will have chosen where to have your baby, what antenatal education you are doing and who you wish to support you through the birth – these are still critical parts of a birth plan even if you don't think you have one because you haven't written it down!

Birth is a powerful thing. It affects us on many levels. It has physical impact and emotional impact. How we feel about our birth can affect so much, from how we feel as a mother, how we feel towards our baby, how we feel about our body, how we are able to feed our baby, and much more. It isn't just a hurdle to be overcome, it does matter. And for something that matters so much, it is something worth thinking about in advance.

It is never too early to start thinking about your birth plan, but it you start researching it at around the start of the third trimester, it should give you time to look into your choices, and to research, discuss and prepare.

'When our baby was born at home without any medical professionals present, it was a great example of why having a plan was important, even when everything doesn't quite go "to plan".

The techniques for labour that I had planned and practised to use, were so important for it being the great experience it was. They kept me calm and focused, even when I realised our baby would be born before the midwife arrived.

When things went off plan, the fact we had a plan meant we had a steer for what we needed to do/request to get things back on course when appropriate. When I was told: "we will just clamp your cord", I could reply saying: "actually I want it left unclamped until after the placenta has been birthed."

When all the professionals descended into the house, being noisy and turning on the lights, we were able to usher them into another room and get the quiet, dark, environment back, allowing the hormones to work to achieve our natural third stage, and protecting that golden hour after birth.

In the absence of a plan, it would have been easy to get carried away down another path, which would have changed the whole experience.' – **Steph and Dean**

case study

His

When it comes to a birth plan, many men feel, at first, as though it's something that doesn't have much to do with them; birth is something their partner goes through, so surely it is her preferences which matter? While this is true, it is still important to get involved for the following three key reasons:

1. Birth impacts on what happens after the birth, on the relationship and on the bond with your baby and each other (see page 217).
2. Showing interest in the birth plan, and supporting your partner can only be positive for your relationship.
3. If you are going to be the birth partner, a key part of your role is to try and support, as far as is reasonably possible, the birth plan to be respected. It follows that you can only fulfil this role if you have a plan to work with!

A birth plan is your opportunity to express preferences for the birth. This doesn't mean it is inflexible; choices made may change depending on how things progress, how your partner is feeling, or other circumstances beyond your control. However, recognising that plans sometimes need to adapt does not mean it is better not to have given it any consideration.

There is value in the process of writing a plan together; you will greater understand the wide range of choices open to you both.

If you plan to be the birth partner, a birth plan is an incredibly useful tool for your role as advocate (see page 105). It makes sense that in order to be able to put forward the birth plan, you need to know and understand it. The added bonus you have is that you alone really know your partner. You have had time to discuss with her the birth preferences, and understand what motivates them. Your midwife is likely to have just met you for the first time, and you can be a great support to helping him/her understand what you want from the birth.

While anyone can read a preference from a piece of paper, if you have worked through the preferences with your partner, you know the relative importance of each one. If you have discussed the plan with your partner, you also are likely to have a better understanding of what alternatives might be preferable if one preference can't be accommodated. For example, if your partner has on her birth plan that she wants to use a birth pool at the local hospital but it is already in use by someone else when you arrive, you are well placed to have an understanding of what a good alternative might be, as you have discussed that part of the plan in detail as you prepared it together. You could then advocate to use a room with a bath or shower attached, or ask to use a room on the midwife led unit were there might be mats and room to move around, or to ask for a birth ball instead.

In labour, your partner will be busy focusing on dealing with the contractions and isn't in the best place to be having long discussions – which is why the birth partner is so crucial, and why birth preferences should be worked on together.

If your preferences do not match your partners, you need to wholeheartedly get on board with her preferences, to ensure there is no friction in the lead up, or during the birth. It is crucial that she can trust you to protect her wishes, as if there is any uncertainty or tension, this can lead to her producing adrenalin during labour which can cause labour to become more difficult.

Get Together

B y writing your birth preferences out together, you will gain an understanding of how you both feel about different options. You have time now to really research and look at the choices from different angles. This is crucial for both of you, mum and birth partner.

Communication is vital as you progress through your journey into parenthood. Exploring your birth preferences together is a great way to practise understanding each other's point of view. Find out what is important to your partner, what they hope for, and if they are worried about anything.

You might be tempted to complete your birth plan by downloading a template or filling in a birth plan preference tick box in your maternity notes. If you feel this adequately covers everything you wish to highlight, then this is fine. However, these are often very limited in their scope as they are generic, and so they may not be worded in the way you would word them, or they may miss aspects which are important to you. Your birth plan, like your birth, is unique to you, so you can create it anyway you wish.

We would suggest, to make sure your birth plan reflects your wishes, once you have both researched and are happy with your preferences, just write them out clearly, concisely and in a logical order – that is now your birth plan.

What are the key choices for your birth plan?

To help your discussion, work through the following together and also do your own further research. Try to explore each choice with an open mind and consider possibilities that you might, at first, assume are not for you. A lot of what we think we know about birth is learnt from TV or hearsay; when we look at evidence we can be surprised that it is contradictory to our beliefs. You might make the same choices after your research, but you open up your possibilities by being prepared to consider a range of options rather than go with assumptions.

Key options to consider include:

- Where do you want to give birth?
- Who will be the birth partner/s?
- What do you want to use in your birth (equipment, techniques)?
- How do you feel about induction?
- What about pain relief?

- Any preferences in positions and mobility for labour and birth?
- What happens after your baby is born?

Where to give birth?

One of the first decisions you will make about your birth is *where* you plan to birth your baby. This is a crucial part of your birth plan which can be overlooked as it is at the very start of the pregnancy and the booking in appointment that you will have been asked where you and your partner plan to give birth. If you change your mind about this at some point in the pregnancy, this is absolutely fine. The initial decision you made then, does not have to be one which you stick to. Experience and research through the pregnancy may mean you feel more comfortable somewhere else. If you and your partner feel like this, ask your midwife to change your place of care.

Up until the 20th century, most babies in the UK were born at home. Nowadays, fewer than 3 per cent are, despite the fact that studies show that home birth is as safe as hospital births for low-risk pregnancies.

Babies themselves can also decide their place of birth! There are always stories of babies arriving in a car or at a supermarket – this certainly makes for an interesting entry on the birth certificate!

There are three main choices when it comes to planning a place of birth: home birth, birth centre or hospital birth (either on a delivery suite or a midwife-led unit). Depending on where you live, you may also have the choice of not just one, but several, hospitals.

It is also not unusual if you don't both initially agree on where you want to have your baby. It is helpful to try and put personal preferences aside and find out what the research shows to help you make an informed decision either way which you both agree on.

Look at the pros and cons of each birth place. Look at the evidence over the assumptions, and work out what offers what you want as a couple. Where will you feel cared for, comfortable and safe? Where fits with your image of the birth you would like to have?

Who should be the birth partner?

Deciding who will be the birth partner is a key part of your birth plan; it is important that a woman feels that she has a person, or people, with her who will enable her to feel as relaxed and cared for as possible.

Today, over 90 per cent of dads in the UK are at the births of their children. Many describe it as an awesome experience, but despite these high statistics, it might not be the right choice for every couple. Some women choose to have a sibling, friend or parent as birth partner. Others choose to hire a doula, who is trained to provide emotional and practical support to a woman in labour. A doula can act as birth partner alongside dad, or in the place of dad. There are lots of choices.

Many men question whether they will be a good birth partner, and may feel nervous about it. Being a birth partner is a responsibility, and it can feel intimidating. Being anxious about something doesn't mean that you are not capable; in fact, it shows that you understand that it is important and want to make sure you do it justice. Making sure that dad feels as prepared as possible and has learnt what to expect will make a big difference (see page 139).

Talk to each other about the role of the birth partner. What do you both see the role as being about? How you do both feel about it? Who do you both want to be there?

Is there anything you want to use at the birth?

While you might not be able to control everything which happens during labour or birth, a key element of your birth preferences is to think about the practical and tangible things that you CAN plan. For the midwives who will be at your birth, it is helpful for them to know what kind of birth you would like them to support you to have and what kind of techniques or environment you are planning which you want their support with.

If you and your partner have been learning a particular approach, such as breathing techniques or positions you want to use, mention that you would like support to use these on your birth plan. This helps the midwife to encourage you both with your techniques, as otherwise they won't know you have these skills to hand!

Think about whether you want dimmed lighting, music playing, people to speak quietly; these are all things you can control about the labour. Spend time thinking about the proactive things you know you can do, which in turn will aid the chances of you both having the birth you want.

Note down if you would like to use a birth pool, bath or shower. Think about your alternatives if it is not available on the day.

Some things you write down may be preferences which are not guaranteed – like using a birth pool – but it is important they are on there too. Yes it can be disappointing if not every preference we wish for comes true, but we can only even have the option of having something if we are first prepared to ask for it.

Talk to each other about what you want to use to manage during labour. Any natural coping methods like breathing practice or relaxation, mindfulness or hypnosis techniques? Any equipment like birthing pools, birth balls, birth stools or your own special pillow? Any preferences on environment, such as music, light, scent, clothing? What you are doing to prepare/practise now to use these skills to their full effect? Is your antenatal education building your confidence in how to use these methods effectively and how they work?

How do you feel about induction of labour?

Induction of labour means kick-starting labour, rather than letting it start of its own accord. This may be offered when medical professionals believe it is safer for mum and baby to birth earlier. It can also be often offered if labour has not started by itself, or soon after, the estimated due date.

Induction is a common intervention, and because it happens before labour begins, sometimes parents miss it off their birth plan. Statistics show that, depending on your hospital, up to 32 per cent of labours are now induced. However, as it can massively impact on how the birth unfolds and some of the choices available, it is important to see it as part of your birth choices and to think in advance about how you feel about it. NICE Guidance acknowledges that there is an increased likelihood of requiring pain relief and an assisted delivery with induction. In first time parents, there is also some evidence which suggests a correlation between induction and higher rates of caesarean section.

Induction is a complex topic and we discuss this further in Chapter 19. Read that chapter alongside your own research as part of your birth plan preparation and discussion together.

Discuss together what induction includes and how you feel about the benefits and risks. Discuss the various circumstances under which induction might be offered, and whether you feel differently about it in different circumstances. Look at the alternatives to induction and how you feel about them. Look at the potential impact induction can have on your birth plan and birth outcomes. Consider how you feel about routine induction (the stretch and sweep) (see page 196) being offered at 40 weeks. Research the Bishop's Score (see page 188) and how you can use this to make decisions about induction.

What are your choices about pain relief?

Labour and birth feel different for every woman, and many things impact the sensations that might be felt during labour.

The preparation you both do, the birth environment created, and choices you make on the day all have an impact. Not knowing how labour will feel can make setting preferences about pain relief difficult, so having as many options as possible to try can be a useful approach.

If there are things which you definitely want, or need to avoid, in terms of pain relief, note these down in your birth plan. If you want to avoid using medicalised pain relief, think about what you will use instead and how you will build your confidence in your method before the big day. Labour can be likened to running a marathon, and so like a marathon, preparation is really important!

Options for pain relief include:

- **Natural techniques for minimising pain.** Attend specialist antenatal classes that help you learn skills and techniques. Research how to use water, such as in a birth pool.

- **Medical pain relief.** This includes TENS machines, which you can hire yourself, to options you will need to access through your midwife such as Entonox, pethidine and epidural.

Pain relief is another complex topic and it is well worth researching the pros and cons of each option as part of your birth plan preparation.

Discuss together the pain relief options and how you feel about them. What are their relative benefits and risks? If you wish to avoid medical pain relief, discuss what alternatives you would like to try and how you are building these into your birth preparations. If you are certain you wish to use medical pain relief, consider what you might use if there is a wait to be able to access this, for example, if an anesthetist is not immediately available.

What about preferences for positions and mobility during labour and birth?

100 years ago, birth moved from home to hospital, and with it came the habit of women laying on their backs in hospital

beds to give birth. However, in the thousands of years before this, and today in countries where women don't routinely give birth in hospitals, this is not the position used. Quite simply, it doesn't aid the birth progress, and left alone, the vast majority of the time, it is not a position anyone would instinctively take up.

While you may not know in advance what position will be most comfortable until it is all happening, it is helpful to consider the options, and even try them out in advance so they don't feel completely alien. You could try standing, kneeling, sitting on or leaning over a birth ball, sitting on a birth stool, sitting on the toilet (yes, really!), all-fours or squatting.

Discuss together what positioning you would like to try during labour, both for the contractions and for birthing. http://dad.info/expecting/birth/helping-at-the-birth-what-can-you-do/

What about after the birth?

Your birth plan shouldn't stop at the birth of your baby; the moment your baby arrives, there are lots of choices to be made!

You might like to give thought to: birthing the placenta, delayed cord clamping, what to use to clamp the cord, holding baby skin-to-skin, whether to give vitamin K, what to do with the placenta, what tests and checks for your baby you would like, and when. You might also like to give some thought as to the environment for the first hour or two after birth. We look in more detail at these choices in Chapter 20.

Discuss together what the options are in the first hour or so after birth. What will your baby be offered and what are the pros, cons and alternatives? What kind of environment do you want for your baby for the first hour as they adjust to the outside world?

Make a few copies of the birth plan, to prevent the possibility of it going missing. Place copies in your birth bags when you pack them. Ideally, you can give a copy to your midwife, and keep a copy as spare or for your own use.

Having a positive birth experience does not require every aspect of the birth plan to become reality, but having a guide to help shape it can make a big difference.

case study

CHAPTER 13

Where should we give birth?

Choosing where to give birth is a really important part of your birth plan, as where you give birth does affect your birth experience. The choices you have depend on your preferences, any medical needs, what is available where you live, and how far you are prepared to travel for the birth.

Hers

Wherever you choose, it should feel right for you and your birth. NICE (National Institute for Health and Care Excellence) support your right to be able to make an informed decision about where to give birth, and highlights that you should have choices.

In weighing up each of the options available to you, try and consider:

- What are the experiences and feedback of other parents who have used the places you are considering?
- What do the statistics show for the level of interventions and types of birth for each place? Remember, that these will

vary between hospitals too, so look into the rates of each individual one.

- Is there easy access to equipment you want to use, such as birth balls, birth pools, etc.?
- How busy is it? What is the ratio of midwives to women in labour? How likely is it that you might be turned away in labour?
- How far away is it? How long will it take to get there?
- Can your partner stay with you after the baby has arrived, or does the birth place have a policy of restricting access?
- Plus any other questions that are important to you; we all have different things that matter to us.

Ultimately, the best place for you to have your baby in is somewhere that you feel safe, comfortable and relaxed.

His

Supporting your partner to explore where she thinks she will feel safest in labour and birth is a really important part of your role. There are probably more choices open to you than you realise, and it's important to research them all, as the place of birth really matters.

You are both likely to have an immediate feeling about where you want to give birth, although whether they are the same feelings or not is another matter! Regardless, it is still a good idea to consider all of your options to make sure it is an informed choice. You might still make the same decision in the end but you might also find out about an option you didn't even know existed, or change your mind on an option that you previously had very strong ideas about.

'When we were planning our birth, my wife mentioned having a home birth, and I automatically said no. I just felt it was a bad idea, even though I had no experience of one. What if something went wrong? Wouldn't it be messy? And noisy?

As time went by, she said it was still important to her, so we researched it a bit more and even went to a home birth information workshop. I learnt a lot about the role of the midwife and how she would be keeping us safe, and advising us if she felt there was a potential problem.

We ended up having a home birth, and it was amazing! Nothing like all the negatives I originally had been imagining! I can't believe I nearly let my preconceptions about what it would be like stop us having that experience.' – **Tom**

case study

Your role in looking at a place of birth is very much in a supporter role. Ultimately, your partner needs to choose the place she feels safest, even if it isn't your preference. This matters because, as you will see in chapter 12 for labour and birth to progress easily and naturally, the environment around the woman in labour is crucial. She has to feel comfortable and safe; if she doesn't then there is a much increased likelihood of intervention or complication.

However, you are also a key part of the birth environment, and if you are feeling very uncomfortable or anxious being in a certain environment, it is possible that your partner will also pick up on this which can affect how safe she feels. So an essential part of your preparation needs to be becoming comfortable with the place she chooses. So, if she wants to be in hospital and you don't like hospitals for whatever reason, what can you do to help ease that? A tour or a virtual tour to try and support you to feel more comfortable? What could you take with you to help you feel more at ease there?

If your partner chooses a home birth and you are uncomfortable about it because of safety, noise, mess, other children or whatever reason, look at statistics and read the experiences of others to get a feel for what it is really like.

If you feel that you can't deal with any issues you have over the place she feels safest to birth, this is something important to discuss with her in advance so that you can discuss other options, like having more than one birth partner present.

From your point of view, it can also be helpful to think about the dad-friendliness of some of the options, so you can have that as part of the discussions.

Find out whether you can stay with your partner after the birth, if needed to. Many fathers find having to leave their new family behind to drive home and come back the next day incredibly difficult and heart wrenching. Similarly, mums value their partner's support and want to have those first special hours together as a family unit.

If your partner has an uncomplicated birth and wishes to, she may go home within a few hours of the birth and not stay overnight. If she does stay overnight, whether you are able to stay with her and your baby will depend on the hospital policies.

An increasing number of hospitals now allow partners to stay overnight, either on a reclining chair on the postnatal ward, or even a camp bed if your partner is in a single room. Birth centres are more likely to be able to accommodate you staying over with your partner; some have double beds that you can share after the birth. Individual hospital and birth centre policies and facilities do vary, often due to space, so do your research and work out what provides the kind of access you both feel suits your family.

In some ways, home-birthing is the most dad-friendly way to birth, as when it is all finished, it is the midwives who leave, not you!

Get Together

Deciding where to give birth is a crucial part of your birth plan. Where you choose to birth can impact on the choices and facilities available to you, as well as who might look after you during labour and birth. Place of birth can also affect the likelihood of having a specific kind of birth so it is helpful to really explore the options. The aim is to choose the place that feels right to you as a family, and every family is different.

Work through the following choices of birth environment together, exploring the pros and cons of each one. Look at which environment will best support you to achieve the birth you wish to have. If you are certain you would like an epidural, then perhaps planning a home birth is not the option for you. If you would like to give birth with minimal intervention, then a home birth might give you the best opportunity to achieve this.

As part of this decision-making process, be sure to really examine any beliefs you already hold about each place of birth to see if they are factually true, or just preconceived assumptions. Sometimes we limit options based on assumption, not even exploring an option because we have already written it off. While we still might make the same choice in the end, by removing assumptions and looking at the facts, we allow ourselves to have more choices to choose from.

Home birth

So what is a home birth? Well, it's exactly that – giving birth to your baby at home. Midwives will come to your house for the birth, bringing with them any equipment they may need.

It is not unusual to feel that the hospital is the safest place to have a baby or to worry about mess or noise. One thing to bear in mind is that midwives are specialists in normal birth; don't underestimate the skills they have! If your midwife thinks there is anything indicative of a problem, they will advise you and recommend moving to hospital. It is incredibly rare that things go wrong in birth without warning signs, and part of the midwife's role is to look out for signs, and take action if any arise. The main reason women are transferred from a planned home birth into hospital is because they ask for additional pain relief which cannot be given at home, rather than any kind of emergency.

One way to look at it: for the majority of labours that start spontaneously, a large part of the birth is likely to be exactly the same as a home birth! You will be at home for most of labour, even if you are planning to birth in the hospital or birth centre. The main difference is that when labour really gets going, you stay put rather than change environments.

If you are concerned about needing pain relief during a home birth, there is the option of using gas and air or pethidine during labour. An epidural cannot be administered at home. If mum decides she wants an epidural, the midwife will just arrange to move the birth to hospital instead – you do not have to stay at home if you change your mind!

If you want labour without medical pain relief, evidence shows you are more likely to achieve this at home than in hospital.

At home you can choose whether or not to hire or buy a birth pool. You can get very sturdy inflatable pools that you can assemble and fill within an hour, so it doesn't have to take up lots of space while you are waiting for baby to arrive. If using water for your birth is an important part of your birth plan, this is a great way to make sure you have the best chance to use it, rather than finding out someone else is in the pool at the hospital.

If for whatever reason, even during labour, you change your mind about giving birth at home, you can! It is no problem at all to just decide to go to the hospital instead, and you don't need to justify why you have changed your mind. Planning for a home birth arguably gives you the easiest opportunity to make your birth place decision on the day, when you know how you feel, rather than trying to guess in advance.

While it is easier to gain the support from your local health trust for a home birth if your pregnancy is low risk, a higher risk pregnancy does not automatically mean it is not an option for you. Where you choose to give birth is your choice, and if at home feels like the right choice for you, discuss it with your midwife. You can also speak to the Supervisor of Midwives at your local hospital to discuss how they can support you, as well as any other options open to you. Some hospitals have a dedicated home birth team, and this can offer a lot of information and support.

Birth centre

In some areas of the UK you may have access to a birth centre. A birth centre is midwifery-led, and can be the middle-ground between birthing at home and going into the medicalised environment of a hospital.

A birth centre offers an environment and support specifically dedicated to birth – it will not be medicalised like a hospital and will aim to provide a 'home away from home' environment, helping you both feel calm, relaxed and confident throughout labour and birth.

Birth centres do vary, so do your research and find out what it offers. There will often be good access to using equipment like a birth pool, birth stools, birthing balls and so forth. Usually, there will also be better opportunities for fathers to be able to stay overnight with their new family.

Similar to a home birth, it also is more likely you will have a straightforward vaginal birth, and not require interventions or more medicalised pain relief.

At a birth centre, you will not be able to access an epidural, although other forms of pain relief will still be available.

If you need specialist care, or there are any concerns about labour, you would be transferred to the nearest hospital maternity unit by ambulance.

Hospital birth

If you choose to birth in hospital, that isn't quite the end of the decision making, as you also have the choice of which hospital. Don't assume that it doesn't really matter which hospital you choose, or that it's just best to go to the nearest one – there are several considerations to look at when making your choice, including:

- What are the experiences and feedback of other parents using it?
- What are the rates for assisted birth and caesarean sections? If you want to increase the likelihood of having a natural birth, then choose a hospital where this is more likely to be achieved statistically. A great website which enables you to compare hospitals maternity statistics is www.birthchoiceuk.com
- Does it have access to facilities you may want to use in birth, such as a birth pool? How many are available? If there is only one of something, the odds are higher that it won't be available on the day you want it.
- Does it have midwife-led birthing rooms as well as a delivery suite?

- How far away the hospital is, and how long will it take to get there at different times of day; the middle of night can very different from rush hour!

Even once you have narrowed it all down and decided that a) you want a hospital birth, and b) which hospital you wish to use, there may still be additional choices to make! Many hospitals now split their birthing facilities into a delivery suite and a midwife-led unit.

Delivery suite usually consists of medicalised birth rooms, with hospital beds and the usual hospital equipment. However, it is helpful to be aware that just because the rooms have beds in them, does not mean that you have to lay in one to give birth! It is still a choice to use equipment like birth balls and to stay mobile in these rooms. Even if mum is being monitored or on a drip, this does not preclude sitting on a birth ball or using positions like all fours or kneeling.

Midwife-led units offer birthing rooms which are usually less medicalised than delivery suite, although how homely they are varies dramatically. They often promote and give access to choices like birth pools, are less likely to have a bed in the room, and are more likely to be furnished with things like beanbags, birth stools, birth couches, and so forth.

To most easily access a midwife-led facility for birth, your pregnancy would need to be considered a 'low risk'. However, even if it is not, this does not mean that automatically you cannot use the facility. If your pregnancy is classed as 'higher risk' and has been under the care of a consultant but you both would like to use the facilities of a midwife led unit, you should both talk to the consultant about it. The consultant may support your wishes to use the facilities – you don't know if you don't ask! It is important to have cleared it and confirmed in your notes before labour begins though as they are unlikely to be around when you go into labour to personally give it the thumbs up – so it is an important aspect of your birth plan to consider.

Discuss together:

What kind of birth do we want to have? What environment best matches to helping us achieve this?

What are the options in the area we live in?

What feels like the right choice for us at this time?

Do we want to change the choice we originally made at our booking in appointment?

CHAPTER 14

What happens in labour?

To support the woman's body to labour and birth as easily as possible, understanding how the body works is pretty important. There is a lot happening simultaneously in the birthing process – muscles working, hormones flowing; having a good oversight of this will really support both mum and birth partner in being able to continue to help things along!

Hers

Labour basically means the body working to give birth, first to your baby, and then the placenta.

You uterus is the incredible organ where your baby spends nine months growing and developing. It grows over 1,000 times in size during pregnancy, and is covered in incredibly powerful muscles. Contractions are the movements of these muscles as the uterus works to birth your baby.

At the bottom of the uterus is the cervix. This is closed during pregnancy to keep baby in, and infection out. During labour, the cervix will gradually open.

Oxytocin is the hormone that gets labour going and keeps it progressing. Oxytocin likes quiet, dark, safe and private environments. The kind of birth environment which you most easily birth in is one where you feel completely uninhibited.

The other hormone you need to know about is Adrenalin. Adrenalin is caused by fear, anxiety, fatigue and feeling uncomfortable or being watched. Adrenalin neutralises Oxytocin, therefore if it is produced in labour, can stall it, stop it and even make it a more painful experience.

How do I know labour has started?

This is different for every woman, and even if you have given birth before, it doesn't mean your experience will be exactly the same as previously. Helpful signs that things may be underway include:

- **A bloody show.** This is mucus from the vagina which is often tinged with blood. It is possible to experience a show days, or weeks, before labour begins so it is not a sure-fire indicator things will happen soon. Conversely, it is also completely possible that you may only have a show near the end of labour. You may also have one and never notice, for example, if you go to the loo in the middle of the night and do not notice.

- **Your waters break.** This is when the amniotic fluid around the baby is released. Thanks to the movies, a huge number of people think this is the key sign that labour is starting. In reality though, waters break at lots of different points in labour, and they most commonly release when labour is very well advanced, and you have already been experiencing contractions.

- **Contractions.** This is a key sign for working out what is happening. In late pregnancy, it is common to get practise contractions which can cause confusion as you try to work out whether things are beginning or not. If you experience contractions that continue if you change position or move around, it may be a sign of the beginning of labour. Contractions begin in different ways for different people; some get a slow, gradual build up, others go straight into a regular, strong pattern.

What are contractions like?

Contractions will feel different to different people, there is a spectrum of labour sensation and this is shown in studies too. Some people report pain (of varying levels), some people say they are just uncomfortable, some people feel little to nothing at all!

How contractions feel can also differ, from tightening sensations, to pressure sensations, to aching sensations.

Where they are felt can also differ, from different places in the abdomen, to lower around the pelvis, to more in the back.

Even if you have had a baby before, there are no givens about how your birth will feel, as each is a unique event.

Will I moo like a cow?

You might do. You might make other noises. Or you might make no noise. It is impossible to know in advance, as all woman are different, and each birth will be different. Sounds made in labour are involuntary, and are just what your body needs to do. Don't worry about being embarrassed; midwives have heard it all before. If you can feel comfortable enough to let go and allow your body to do what it needs to do, you will be supporting your labour to happen as it needs to.

What if I poo myself?

Many women worry about this, so if the thought has crossed your mind, you are not alone! As baby moves down to be born, the pressure can cause an emptying of the bowel. Although it might seem mortifying to you now, midwives looking after you will not be at all bothered and will have seen it many times before. A midwife will just clean anything away. In one way, your midwife will see it as a great thing to happen, as it signals that baby is moving in the right direction!

Just because you might feel as though you need a poo, it doesn't mean that you will. As baby moves down, the sensation can feel the same as pooing, but actually it is just baby that you can feel. Being able to relax and go with the sensation is important, as that's what you need to do to birth your baby. If you are trying to resist what feels like having a poo, then you may be holding your baby in and prolonging your labour.

This is one of the reasons that many women spend some time labouring on the toilet; it is a place where they feel more comfortable with these kinds of sensations, where they have some privacy, and can just allow their body to work.

If you are in a birth pool and you have a poo, the midwife will just scoop it out with a small net or sieve. This is so common that they will always have one to hand!

What is 'transition'?

At the end of the first stage of labour, when the cervix is finishing dilating and baby is ready to make the final part of their journey, some women experience 'transition'. Not all women do, but if you do, it can be the point where you can feel a real loss of control. Understanding in advance what is happening won't prevent it, but can help you keep it in perspective if it does occur.

During transition, a surge of adrenalin floods the body. This is all part of Mother Nature energising you ready for the final push, and waking you up to receive your baby!

The adrenalin surge can cause you to shake; jiggling legs or shivering is common. It is also possible to feel nauseous or vomit. Emotionally, all of that adrenalin can send you into a 'fight or flight' mode, which is often known as the 'self-doubt phase'. Even the calmest woman at this point may start saying things like: *'I can't do it'*, or *'I want a caesarean'*; you may even try to leave the room!

There is some suggestion that the more relaxed and 'in the zone' a woman has been in, the less likely this adrenalin surge will cause her to feel these feelings.

What position should I give birth in?

Some positions will make giving birth easier, and others more difficult. Despite what has been commonly depicted on TV, birthing on your back makes it much more difficult. Your pelvis is designed to be mobile during birth (the hormone Relaxin produced in pregnancy relaxes the ligaments of the pelvis) and so it is able to stretch and open. Your tailbone is designed to move backwards as your baby moves down through the pelvis; if you are laid on the tailbone during birth, it cannot move as fully as it is designed to do, so your baby has to be birthed through a small space, making it more difficult.

The birth canal curves upwards at the vagina, in an 'L' shape. This means that as your baby reaches the corner of the L, you are working against gravity to birth them if you are on your back.

There is also an increased risk of perineal damage, as birthing in this position causes baby's head to come more strongly into contact with the perineum than it would in a more upright position.

All that said, the 'right' birthing position is the one which feels right to you on the day.

Positions that can make this stage a little physiologically easier include kneeling or being on all-fours. If you don't feel like you can bear your weight, or you are tired, lying on your side will still allow pelvis mobility (as you will not be lain on your tailbone, so it will be able to move backwards), and your position, while not harnessing gravity, will not be going against it.

You don't have to change position between labour and birth; if you are in a comfortable position, stay where you are, your midwife will be able to support you.

His

If you want to support your partner during the birth of your baby, it is important to have a basic understanding of what is happening in her body during the process. Read the HERS section of this chapter to gain an insight into all this. It is crucial that you do this, as you do need to have an understanding of how her body works and what it will be doing, in your role of supporting that.

The key for you is to understand how to support your partner during labour and birth, using this knowledge. The next two chapters, 'The birth partner' and 'Practical tips for birthing' will give you practical advice on how you can help during labour and birth.

Make sure you also spend time supporting your partner to write a birth plan (see page 110). It is crucial to write a birth plan so that you have time to research all the different options available to you, including where to have your baby, how you would like to manage labour, and your choices for your baby in the first minutes of his or her life.

Get Together

As the body goes through changes during birth, you will also often experience changing behaviours and instincts which accompany those too. These can be unfamiliar to both of you, and the key is to stay working together through them.

What do you expect?

To help you prepare for what you might experience, discuss some of the following behaviours which might happen during birth, and how you could work together through each of these. What can/should the birth partner do to support mum physically or emotionally if she is:

- Making noises?
- Wants to be upright?
- Wants privacy?
- Is very quiet?
- Is feeling afraid?
- Needs to keep moving around?
- Feels very worn out?
- Doubts her abilities?

Staying mobile?

Labour and birth are physical acts, and there are some physical positions which make it easier or harder for our bodies to undertake them. Being upright is shown in numerous studies to make birthing easier. An upright position increases space in the pelvis by up to 30 per cent which obviously means more room for baby to pass through, meaning an easier and quicker birth (see page 116).

Talk together in advance about which positions mum might want to use during labour, and how you can work together to support her to use those positions. If she finds standing upright helpful in labour, how can you as birth partner support her to stay standing when she is more tired? Or working through a strong contraction?

Labour sensations and contractions, often make women feel like they are unable to keep still, wanting to move will be instinctive. Working with her body, instead of against it, helps the body and baby birth. Changing position, swaying the hips, walking and leaning forward are all common and can help the baby get into a good position and labour to progress. Discuss together that if she finds moving around in labour helpful, how can you support this? Where could you both walk together in early labour? What about when things are more intense? Have you practiced back massage together as she rocks on a birth ball to know whether that might work?

Change your mind?

All women are different during labour, some make loud noises, some are almost silent. Sometimes the noises that she makes (or doesn't make!) may make the birth partner worry. We discuss in the next chapter why it is important that a birth partner does not make assumptions, and leap in with a desire to 'fix it' which could actually be detrimental to the birth (see page 143).

Sometimes women vocalise as a part of fear or tension release. She may say things which are not really true, but as her body is working to release her baby, she may also be saying things as part of also releasing feelings. Not everything a woman says in labour is necessarily how she really feels or what she wants. Women can also be overcome with self-doubt, and reassurance can be really important in helping her decide if something she is suddenly asking for is really what she wants, or it was a blip of fear.

'I remember telling my husband that I did not want to do it any more. I told him I wanted an epidural and for it all to stop. The next moment my midwife told me that I was 6cm dilated and I could use the birth pool if I wanted. Wow, what a difference knowing that I had progressed made me feel, and the feeling of the water as I got in the pool was amazing! I hadn't really wanted an epidural, but saying I did just felt like my way of signalling to everyone that I was finding it harder and needed some help. I was so glad I didn't have one, as my daughter was born 40 minutes later and it was everything I had hoped for.' – **Bethany**

case study

There may, however, come a point where mum truly wishes to deviate (for whatever reason) from the original birth plan you prepared together. It can be difficult therefore, for a birth partner to work out whether it is time to reassure and keep mum on track, or to advocate for her and her changed wishes!

If you want to be sure that during labour you are able to communicate between you (without confusion or doubt) a change from the plan, code word is a handy tool you can use. So decide together a code word now – pick something between yourselves which is easy to remember but you wouldn't use in everyday conversation. Make sure you both are very clear on which word you have chosen and how you will use the code word technique in labour.

The agreement between yourselves is that if in labour mum suggests she wants to deviate from the birth plan, the first time she does so, you will ignore her request and reassure her. This way, if she is just vocalising, you are not overreacting. But if she asks again, take a moment to really connect with her and ask her if she is sure, and ask her for the code word. This gives her a moment to really consider if she definitely wants you to take action and to decide whether to give you the code word.

If she refuses to give you the code word, you know she is just vocalising, and more reassurance or perhaps a change in environment might be helpful.

CHAPTER 15

The birth partner

One of the biggest influences in the birth environment are the people around us and especially our birth partner. Our birth partner is the person who is likely to be with us from very early on in labour right to the end, and therefore can have a huge impact.

Hers

So what is your birth partner there to do? His or her role is to support you in practical and emotional ways during labour and birth. This could be anything from filling the birth pool, driving you to hospital, rubbing your back and giving you positive encouragement. Your partner can hold you through a contraction, help you get changed, bring you something to drink or eat. Their role is to advocate your birth plan and if it looks like things may deviate, to help make sure your wishes, as far as possible, are respected in spite of those changes.

The role of birth partner is sometimes misunderstood. Sometimes I have heard mums-to-be say things to their partner like, 'You will be at the birth so you can see what I have to go through to have our baby' or 'I want you to see the pain I suffer giving birth.' In reality, a birth partner is not there as an observer (in fact we look in Chapter 14 how feeling observed can be counterproductive to labour), but they have an important role in protecting the birth environment and advocating your wishes and preferences.

There is also no reason to think that it will be such a traumatic event they will be witnessing either! In fact, your birth partner can be the key to supporting you to having a more positive labour and minimising pain. Numerous studies have evidenced how the birth partner has the capacity to impact on the length of labour, how much pain is perceived, the likelihood of interventions, of an assisted birth or even a Caesarean birth – and a confident birth partner is much more likely to be able to support you to have a positive labour and birth.

Sometimes we feel the opposite, and we worry that the birth will be difficult for our partner so we seek to work out ways of relieving some of the pressure on them by considering having other birth partners. We have certainly come across this several times in couples where dad has suffered with previous trauma (which may be related to birth, or may be related to other circumstances – for families where dad has served in the military). If this is something which you are considering, remember not to make any assumptions about how your partner feels and talk to them about it first.

Ultimately, if you decide between yourselves that your partner is going to be your sole birth partner, he needs to be prepared for his role and not feel afraid. Supporting them to feel confident about their abilities and not put them down, or assume they won't be capable is crucial.

However, it also helps when they can be prepared, understand what their role is and how to undertake it. By reading this book or going to classes, your husband will be preparing – so try to encourage him, and if he wants to talk about what he has learnt, allow him to do so and focus on his journey. If he doesn't want to, don't force him – let him learn in his own way. Try not to nag him to read it, or tell him off for not reading it enough or quickly, as it can be a bit of a turn off. Positive encouragement is preferable here.

If for some reason, your partner wants to be there but you are concerned he won't be able to fulfil what you need on his own, discuss this with him. Dads can feel worried that if there is someone else there, like your mum, that they will be pushed out and not get those first moments to bond with their child. In these situations, it can be useful to discuss how your wishes for support can be respected, but while also respecting how he feels and how he wants to be involved. It is not uncommon for dads to feel fears during the pregnancy of being pushed out once the baby arrives, so it is just important to be aware of this so you can make sure any decisions you make are done mindfully and sensitively. As usual, communication is the key!

His

S tudies show that a birth partner can have a positive impact upon the length of labour, the degree of pain experienced, and the outcome of the birth. It is definitely not a role to dismiss as unimportant or treat too humorously.

World-renowned birth pioneer Michel Odent argued that such is the influence of the birth partner, that dads should not even be present at the birth. He blamed nervous dads in the delivery room for the increase in caesarean sections. This seems over the top to us, but there are some key truths behind his views: dads can have a very real, and in some cases, detrimental impact on childbirth. We believe that, however, dads who properly prepare and are supported to learn to be best birth partners they can, have a hugely beneficial and positive impact on birth.

In the majority of couples, your partner will want you with her during the birth. You made this baby together and will be raising this baby together, so it makes sense that you now welcome your baby into the world together. But with this comes responsibility; responsibility to be the best support you can be. Preparation for a positive birth experience is not just the domain of the woman.

We break down the role of the birth partner into two key parts:

Role 1: Protector

As we explored on page 130, adrenalin can have a very detrimental impact on labour progress. If you can help your partner to feel safe and 'protected', you will help keep the happy hormone oxytocin flowing, and minimise the production of adrenalin.

How can you do this? Think about how you can make the room feel more relaxing and less medical. Can you dim the lights and play relaxing music? If you spot something in your partner's view that you feel may cause a problem, move it! You can start this at home, during the drive and walking in to the maternity suite. Do you seem relaxed and in control? If your partner tells you that her contractions have slowed walking in to the hospital, it might be a surge of adrenalin neutralising the oxytocin. Reassure her that you will be in a calm, quiet room soon.

You might be surprised to hear that you also need to protect your partner from yourself! During labour, your partner's senses will be heightened; Mother Nature gave this as a gift to labouring women so that they can sense any dangers. These heightened senses mean that your partner will sense any worries or tension coming from you. In a nutshell: she can smell your fear! If she senses you are afraid or worried, it will trigger her fear and thus her adrenalin. The better prepared and informed you are, the calmer and more confident you will be. If you need a reminder, look how calm the midwife is.

Your role is to focus on her and to keep reassuring her. Your job is not to direct, so resist any urge to tell her what to do and to 'coach' her. Your role is to protect; this can be easier said than done for many men due to an inbuilt 'fix-it reflex', however, understanding that you have this impulse is the first step to taking control of it.

The fix-it reflex

Humans feel an impulse to help, and men especially like to seek out practical solutions. When it comes to birth, reigning in this 'fix-it' reflex is actually really important. When your partner appears to be in pain or distress, as in labour, a natural instinct tells us to intervene and get her help. We may do this in a number of ways, such as taking her to the hospital too early (because we want her there, rather than her wanting to be there!), asking her if she wants pain relief, or other interventions. As we become fearful and anxious, your partner begins to pick up on your emotional state, which can stimulate a release of adrenalin in her body, with all the negative consequences that can bring.

Dads, it is not up to you to make these decisions. You have to control your instinct to fix the situation. You have your roles and you should concentrate on those. If your partner does need help, she will ask for it.

It is important to not try to fix things and interfere. For example, the moment you suggest some pain relief because you want to fix things, you have suggested to her that she is not coping. Even if she is coping, she may suddenly feel that you are doubting her. This breaks that protection and trust you are meant to be providing for her. If she doubts herself and becomes anxious, here comes that adrenalin.

It is an admirable quality to want to protect your partner and family. What you need to be aware of is that, at certain points, and during birth being one of them, your fix-it reflex can cause more harm than good. One of the ways you can learn to control this reflex is by being mindful of your role, and be confident in the techniques you will be using as birth partner.

Role 2: Advocate

Put simply, to be an advocate is to make sure your partner's wishes are heard and understood. So common sense should tell you that you cannot advocate successfully if you don't know what your partner's wishes are. If you wait until she is in labour, she may not be able to tell you how she feels, so making the birth plan (see page 105) together is so important.

If you find a topic that you do not see eye-to-eye on, then your partner's wishes come first. You have to wholeheartedly accept this; a true advocate always puts forward the viewpoint of the person they are advocating for, regardless of their own feelings on the matter. It is also crucial for the birth process that your partner has complete trust that you will honour her wishes (see page 109).

Most women when labouring, in the right environment, will 'zone out'. This means that during contractions your partner will almost 'go into herself' and be focused on what she is doing. You need to protect that state. Nobody, not you, not the midwife, should ask her a question during a contraction. If anyone does ask her a question, gently ask the person to wait a moment and re-ask the question when the contraction has passed.

During labour, you partner may be offered pain relief or other interventions. Here, your role as her advocate is to ensure that the wishes that you have discussed are respected. During labour, your partner is vulnerable on two counts: firstly, the logical right side of her brain shuts down which enables her to stay in the birthing zone; this means she cannot easily debate or discuss, and forcing her to do so brings her out of the birthing zone and can impact on her birth experience. Secondly, your partner is vulnerable as she may be finding labour a very challenging experience; this may make her susceptible to agree to things she does not really want, when all she really needs is encouragement and support.

Safeguarding your partner's wishes is your job. You may need to explain her preferences, you need ensure these are respected, and that she isn't pressured into anything she isn't comfortable with. For any treatment, it will be your partner who will ultimately need to consent/or not consent. She is classed as the 'patient', but you can certainly back her up and reaffirm her wishes at each step, and this is absolutely crucial.

If after attending classes and reading as much as you can, you come to the conclusion that you don't feel you can fulfil everything your partner needs of a birth partner, that is okay; you mustn't feel pressured into it. You also deserve to be able to have a positive experience too. If you do feel this way, discuss it with your partner, and explain how you feel. Explain how it is not that you do not want to be there, but you want her to have the very best support and you are not sure you are able to provide it.

Support your partner to find someone who will fulfil the role, so that she doesn't feel that you are disinterested. Keep talking and working together; choosing to not be at the birth doesn't mean that you still cannot support in a multitude of other ways. You can still support the birth plan, attend antenatal classes and so forth. While you may both opt for another birth partner, if circumstances changed and you are there unexpectedly, having some idea of what to expect and do, even on a basic level, will be helpful. It is unlikely to happen, but sometimes things don't go exactly to plan!

Sometimes a woman might decide that she wants more support than she feels her partner can provide, or wishes to have another person there who is important to her. While this may be difficult to hear, it is important to understand that your partner does need to feel comfortable that she has the best support around her, as this will make her birth easier. This does mean that we have to put her wishes before our own. You will always be the father of your baby though, and that is a connection and relationship that is unique, regardless of who else may be at the birth.

Get Together

A key part of your birth planning is asking yourselves who should be the birth partner/s at the birth of your baby? This isn't a question that anyone can answer for you; you need to decide as a couple. There are a number of choices open to you that you can talk through:

- **Dad as the sole birth partner.** This is probably the most usual choice couples make in the UK, but just because it is a popular choice doesn't mean it is necessarily the choice that suits you. Couples can feel under a lot of pressure due to cultural expectations to choose this path, but if you decide it isn't the right choice for you, that is no one's business but your own.

- **Having two birth partners.** Having another supporter alongside dad in the birth room. This could be a family member, friend, doula or private midwife (see below).

- **Having a family member or friend as the sole birth partner.**

- **Hiring a doula.** Doulas are trained to provide support for expectant parents at their birth. They can support you both through the birth, or a doula can be a sole birth partner. You can find out more about the support doulas provide and see a list of those in your local area by visiting www.doulauk.org.

Whatever you both choose, it is important to recognise that it is a choice.

Discuss:

Who do we want at the birth?

What do they need to be able to do?

What can we do to help them prepare to be the best birth partner they can be?

CHAPTER 16

Practical tips for birthing

Once you understand what is happening in the body during labour and birth, thoughts turn to what practical stuff we can do to help keep things moving forwards positively. The good news is there are lots of things you can do, as well lots of things you can also avoid, which will both really make a difference to your birth experience.

Hers

Take your mind off it, and get some rest

When labour begins, try not to focus on it too much. It could take a while to get going properly and over-analysing it can be tiring mentally, and can make it feel like it's been going on much longer than it actually has. Do something relaxing and normal to you: bake, go for a walk, do some gentle exercises on your birth ball, watch something nice on TV (think oxytocin, not adrenalin – so funny, happy films rather than horrors or weepies!). Do these things for as long as feels right.

If contractions begin in the evening or during the night, don't think that you have to stay up or get out of bed; if it is possible to get some rest, get some rest. It may not be the best night's sleep you ever had, but you will be more rested than if you hadn't had it. If the sensations force you out of bed, then listen to your body and move around. If your contractions are still fairly far apart, you may want to go back to bed to rest between them.

Trying to stay up when your body is tired will make your body produce adrenalin (see page 130). When you are relaxed and sleepy your body will produce oxytocin, which can really help your labour. For a first-time pregnancy the early stages of labour can last for many hours. If you spend all evening awake, you will be tired by the next morning which means adrenalin will flood your body to keep you going, thereby slowing down your labour. By the time you might have rested enough to allow the oxytocin to do its thing, it may be the next evening again and you are potentially facing a second night with no sleep!

Focus on your breathing

For the muscles surrounding the uterus (see page 129) to work as effectively and efficiently as possible, they need to be fuelled. And as with any muscle in the body, their fuel is oxygen.

Breathing can also help you cope with your contractions by giving a focus point. Breathing is not a distraction from a contraction, but something positive we can put our focus and energies into, one contraction at a time.

You don't need any 'special' breathing techniques in labour, but it can take a bit of practise to learn how to focus on breathing when there are other distractions around you. Joining a class that will support you to practise tuning in to your breathing can be very beneficial, whether yoga, Pilates or a specific antenatal class, like our MummyNatal classes which include breathing practice each week.

Stay hydrated

Drinking plenty of water during labour is really important, and can affect the pace of your labour and also how it feels. It is not uncommon for women to be so focused in labour that they forget to drink, leading to dehydration. This is compounded if you are breathing deeply through contractions, as you will lose a lot of moisture on your outbreath.

When the body is dehydrated, the muscle output is decreased by 30 per cent. For labour, this means that the uterine muscles will be working just as hard, but will be 30 per cent less effective, so labour can take longer. Dehydration also causes contractions to feel stronger, which can cause increased fatigue and make labour harder to manage. Dehydration can also lead to an increase in body temperature, which may lead to more intervention from professionals.

While staying hydrated is important, so is emptying your bladder! There is only so much space in your body and a full bladder can get in the way of your baby moving downwards in labour; this might cause you discomfort and lengthen how long labour will take. Regular trips to the loo to empty your bladder can be a great way of avoiding this.

Relax your body

Did you know that tension travels? So, if you are tense in one area of your body, then you are not only tense in that area, but that tensions causes changes in other parts of your body too? Furthermore, there is a very strong connection between the jawbone and the pelvis (which are connected via the spine). This means if we are tense in our jaw (so mouth closed, teeth clenched) that that tension is also traveling and manifesting itself in the pelvic area. During birth, as the basic idea is for your baby to travel through your pelvis, so it follows that the more open and relaxed and able to stretch and move to accommodate your baby – the easier it will be, the more your pelvis is closed, and tense and rigid – the harder (and probably more painful) it will be.

So in labour, being able to notice if we are holding tension so we can then have the choice to try and let that tension go, can be really beneficial.

Look for antenatal classes that will teach you how to identify any areas of tension, through techniques like body scanning or breathing practice.

Enjoy the rests between contractions

Women can become very focused on contractions; how it will feel, how long it will be, timing them, will I be able to cope, and so on. It is easy to forget all about the glorious rests we get between each one!

It is a different way of looking at it, but learning to focus and look for the rests, can completely change how you experience your entire labour. Enjoying each rest fully, rather than spending lots of physical and mental energy thinking or worrying about the next contraction is very powerful.

During your rests, by just relaxing and breathing, you will also be replenishing your body with fresh blood flow and oxygen. This helps the uterus work effectively, and the baby to cope well with labour.

Stay at home as long as possible

If you are planning to have your baby in hospital, timing when you travel in can be important. It is common that a change of environment will have some impact on your labour, and can slow it down. If you are in well-established labour, this can usually be overcome quickly; once you settle into your new environment you will settle down and relax. However, in early labour, the impact can be a lot greater, vastly slowing progress and contractions.

Being in hospital can mean there are fewer distractions and home comforts, so time can feel longer. Having midwives checking on you regularly can cause a feeling (often subconsciously, but very powerful nonetheless) of 'performance anxiety'; you might feel you need to get a move on, perform better, that you might be wasting peoples' time, something is wrong, etc. This anxiety can have a negative impact on labour as your body produces adrenalin (see page 130).

In addition, feeling 'observed' can restrict the 'Sphincter Law'. This is the idea that the cervix acts like a sphincter muscle and will only relax to release and open when we feel uninhibited and unobserved. Think about how we don't feel comfortable going to the loo with a lot of strangers watching, and this is the same for birthing. All mammals are designed to want to find a quiet, safe place to give birth. If you are in an environment where you feel uninhibited, it can affect the length of your labour and how it feels. Your cervix will resist opening as your body is signalling it isn't safe, yet your contractions are still trying to pull it open, so this is likely to be more painful.

Get into your 'birth zone'

When labour starts getting more intense you are likely to want to retreat to somewhere that feels safe, so home rather than wandering around the local park. Being in your 'space' will allow the birthing hormones to keep working. If you are having a home birth, you can just stay in your safe place and call the midwife out when you feel ready. If you are having a birth in hospital or a birth centre, stay at home until you feel ready to go in. Keep the lights low, close the curtains, listen to some soothing music and practise any techniques you may have learnt at antenatal classes.

His

It is an amazing experience to hear the words: 'I think labour has started.' All kinds of thoughts and feelings can pass through your mind, and the instant reaction is:

'What do I do?' There is no need to panic. Here's your check-list and action plan:

Check that it is labour!

In the final weeks of pregnancy it is not uncommon for a woman to have warm-up contractions. Your partner may think labour is beginning, and then may find it all suddenly stops. The signs that labour may have started, include:

- Contractions, which continue even when your partner is moving around. Warm-up contractions tend to happen mostly when sitting or lying down, stopping when she moves.
- The amniotic fluid around the baby is released, known as the waters breaking.
- A bloody show (a blood-stained mucus from the vagina). See page 130.

It is important to note that your partner may experience these symptoms and it does not automatically mean that labour has started. Equally, your partner may only experience contractions at first, with no bloody show or waters breaking. Waters often don't break until labour is well underway, despite what you may have seen in the movies.

Should you suspect your partner's waters have broken, but there are no other labour signs, it is a good idea to let your midwife know so mum and baby can be checked to make sure all is ok. If you think the waters have broken and it is before 37 weeks, always seek medical advice.

Time the contractions

Subtly keep an eye on your partner's contractions and note to yourself how frequent they are, how long they are lasting, whether they seem to be getting stronger and if they are settling into a pattern. But don't stand in front of her with a stopwatch like she is an athlete!

You can use an ordinary watch or, if you own a smart-phone, download an app to help you keep track if you like.

Whatever you choose, don't get carried away with exploring all the features of the app or spend the whole time staring at your watch; labours vary, and if your app tells you one thing, but your instincts tell you something else, ditch your phone and listen to those instincts.

Contact your midwife

When the contractions are five minutes apart, and are lasting for about a minute and have been in that pattern for several contractions, phone your midwife or hospital maternity unit.

Run a bath for your partner

Offer to run a nice warm bath for your partner; use the birth pool if you have one at home. Water is a highly effective form of natural pain relief, so if your partner is feeling any discomfort from the contractions, this may help to ease that. Warm water can also encourage labour to progress even more quickly if you are in established labour, and so a bath may support the contractions to become stronger and closer together. So once your partner is in the bath, don't wander far off!

Offer massage

Now is a good time to offer a massage, if you have been learning any techniques. You could gently stroke her arms and back, as this will help her produce endorphins which are the body's natural pain relief. If your partner isn't keen on soft strokes, try holding her hand or firmly rubbing her lower back. Bear in mind over 50 per cent of women are not that keen on being touched while in labour, so don't take it personally if she doesn't like it, and stop if asked.

Both keep hydrated

Make sure you are encouraging your partner to drink. In more advanced labour, you could use those bendy straws from your birth bag (see page 93), and offer her sips between contractions.

Don't forget to drink enough yourself as you need to look after yourself too.

If you're planning a home birth ...

Stay with your partner (if you need to walk the dog or collect a child, ask a friend!) Make your home as comfortable and relaxing as possible while you wait for the midwife to arrive. Dim the lights low, make sure the room is warm or cool enough, and put on some relaxing music. If you have a birth pool, help her to get into that if she feels she would like to.

If you're planning a hospital or birth centre birth ...

Know how long it will take to get there and when you both judge the time is right, off you go! On the journey, you are likely to be feeling exhilarated and anxious. It can be pretty distracting to be the chauffeur for a woman in labour, but drive slowly and calmly as it's important that you all arrive safely. If it is rush hour or you get caught in a traffic jam and are concerned you won't make it in time, you can call 999 for an ambulance.

Park with as little stress as possible; your priority is to keep your partner calm. You can always sort out a parking ticket later, and there is often a system in place for this. If you have difficulty parking then make sure you leave the car somewhere it is not going to get in the way, and get your partner indoors, checking that you have all the birth bags from the car, while keeping her feeling as relaxed as possible.

When you arrive at the hospital ...

Explain to the maternity reception who you are, and when you are introduced to your midwife show her the birth plan.

Labour can often slow down when arriving at hospital, so the more you can reassure and help your partner settle in and relax, the more likely it will resume again quickly.

Active labour and beyond

Now that you have support with you, wherever you are giving birth, keep attending to the needs of your partner and reassuring her. Keep the lights in the room dimmed and have some music gently playing in the background. Tell her how brilliantly she is doing, and how much you love her. Wipe her face with a cold flannel if she is hot and finds it soothing. If you notice her holding her breath, encourage her to breathe and do it with her. Hold her hand or place your hand on her shoulder so that she knows she is not alone.

When baby arrives

This is such an awe-inspiring moment, and one where you can take some time to gaze at the little miracle you have helped create. Remember to get some photos of those first moments!

Your birth partner role is not quite over yet; it is time to think about your birth plan regarding the third stage, cord clamping, vitamin K and so forth.

Then finally you will be able to sit together and enjoy some moments alone as a new family, before you both announce your new baby to the world!

What do I do if the baby comes before the midwife?

It is a common fear of many fathers-to-be that they may not get to the hospital in time, or the midwife might not arrive at their home in time. What if you have to act as midwife to your own partner?

To reassure you, you are far more likely to arrive at the hospital/call the midwife earlier than needed, than have an unexpected home birth. It is also very unlikely for a first pregnancy. However, it does happen occasionally.

Just for your reassurance, if you find yourself in this situation, here are the steps to follow (and most of these are common sense anyway you will see!):

- If you believe that your baby's arrival is imminent and especially if your partner says she is pushing, this is not the time to start a car journey. It's warmer and safer to give birth unplanned at home than at the side of the motorway.

It is also easier for a midwife or medical support to find you at home.

- Call 999. Although having a baby is not a medical emergency, having some support come out to you is important. Tell them clearly that you are at home with no medical support.

- The operator will ask you what is happening and talk you through what you need to do, if anything, while the paramedics are on the way. The operator will stay on the phone the whole time to offer you support and advice, if needed.

- Encourage your partner to be in any position she feels comfortable in. All-fours or kneeling-up are good positions for birthing.

- Just reassure your partner. Tell her to trust her body and to allow it to do whatever it is doing. Stay with her and tell her you are there for her.

- Make sure your front door is unlocked so assistance can come straight in.

- If you see your baby's head emerging, get ready to catch him or her as the shoulders are birthed. Don't touch or tug the baby while emerging. If you can see a loop of cord around your baby's neck (very common, and not usually an issue) you can gently unloop it, but don't pull on the cord.

- When you or your partner have caught your baby, place the baby on mum's chest. This keeps your baby warm and helps to support his or her vital systems. Cover them both with a clean blanket or towel (or whatever you have to hand) to keep them warm.

- Leave your baby attached to the cord; don't try to clamp or cut it. Your baby will still be receiving oxygen via blood from the cord. Birthing the placenta with the cord attached is completely normal.

- If your partner starts birthing the placenta and you are still without medical support, just reassure her and let her body do the work. When the placenta is birthed, just leave it alone; there is still no urgency to clamp or cut the cord. Make sure the 999 operator knows what is happening so they can update the professionals on their way to meet you.

■ Then just wait for someone to arrive to congratulate you! The paramedics will check your partner and baby to make sure all is ok, and you will have a fantastic story to tell for the rest of your lives!

Get Together

As you start to prepare for labour and birth, this is a good time to 'revise' any skills or practices you have learnt in your antenatal preparation, so you are both clear. Can you make time to practise at home, so you are both confident in what you plan to do and how you plan to do it? Practise is most effective when you both do it as you both have a role in making it work.

Try practising a couple of times a week. Mum, how you might use breathing skills, maybe practising in any positions you might use for during and between contractions.

Dad, what can you say or do to reassure and relax mum as she is doing this? How might you support her to use breathing to stay focused? You may also have practical preparations too, like making sure you know how to inflate the birth pool.

While it might seem that this kind of practise is most relevant for mum, it is still important for the birth partner to also practise breathing or relaxation exercises. It is true that it will be mum who uses them to stay focused and calm in labour, but understanding how they work through personal experience, can really enhance how the birth partner can support her by talking her through using the techniques.

More than that, they are also useful skills for birth partners to be able to use for themselves, if they feel any stress or tension during labour. At such an important time in our lives, it is not unusual to have moments of feeling overwhelmed at everything we are seeing and the sense of responsibility and care towards our partner. However, when birth partners are stressed, mums can pick up on it and 'catch' that stress – as we looked at in Chapter 14, women in labour are more sensitive and pick up on things around them more easily. So it can also be helpful for birth partners to be able to use the techniques to stay calm themselves, for their own mental wellbeing, but also to make sure that they are not the ones bringing stress in and negatively affecting labour.

So discuss together what you would like to practise and dedicate a time to doing so together. Maybe you agree on just before dinner twice a week. It doesn't matter, just choose when and make time.

A simple breathing exercise

Take it in turns to read this aloud to each other, to practise the skill of using your breath as a focusing tool. For mum, it can be helpful to do this in a position she is planning to use for labour – so sitting on a birth ball, leaning on a birth ball or back of a chair, etc.

Why not also experiment with your environment each time you practise, to see what helps you both focus better – gentle music in the background, a candle as a focal point, closing the curtains – this is all part of your learning in preparation for birth.

Read this slowly, and gently, pausing at the end of sentences to allow your partner to really follow your guidance and find their focus.

So now we are going to begin our breathing practice, so to allow yourself to truly focus, let your eyes close now, or if that isn't comfortable for you, gaze at a spot in the room in the distance or at the light of the candle in the room.

And you are now going to bring all of your awareness to your breath. Turn your attention now to focus entirely on the action of your breath.

Just completely tuning in and focusing on the repetitiveness of the pattern of taking a breath in, followed by a breath out. Notice the small pauses you naturally place between each breath.

Don't try to control your breath in any way, just allow it to flow however feels natural for you.

Now, notice where you feel your breath. Maybe you feel it in your nose, your throat. Maybe you feel it in the rise and fall of your chest, or your tummy. Where do you feel it most strongly? Allow yourself to really focus there on that sensation now, following the pattern of the in-breath and the out-breath.

As you breathe, can you hear it? Are there any sounds as you breathe in and out? If so, focus on listening to this sound as well, to help you focus.

If you find your mind wandering off, just notice it has happened but choose to leave the thoughts it has wandered to, to one side for a while, and bring your attention back to your breath. Bring your attention back to the aspect of your breath that you find the easiest to focus on – be it where you feel it, the sound, the rhythm.

Feel your breath. Hear your breath. Find calm in its natural, reassuring, repetitive pattern. Use this practice to find out for yourself where you can most strongly tune into your own breathing rhythm to find that sense of focus.

Feel a sense of calm and confidence knowing you can use this practice as a skill to focus yourself any time you need to. Each time you practise, it will become a little easier to focus the next time too.

And when you feel ready, you can open your eyes and finish your practice.

CHAPTER 17

Caesarean birth

There are times when birth by caesarean section is necessary for the wellbeing of mum and/or baby, and this is why we are fortunate in the UK to have access to medical care and professionals.

However, if this is the path your birth takes and it wasn't something you had been prepared for or expecting, you can experience mixed feelings and anxiety. It is often assumed that in a caesarean birth, we will have no power to express any preferences. While there might be instances where our preferences cannot be facilitated, there are often still preferences we can have supported.

Hers

A caesarean section is a surgery whereby an obstetrician makes a cut through your abdomen and uterus, in order to lift your baby out. A caesarean is the most common type of major surgery that women have, and in the UK each year, nearly one quarter of babies are born via caesarean.

An 'elective' caesarean is one which has been planned before labour begins, and takes place on a scheduled date and time. This constitutes about 40 per cent of caesarean births in the UK.

An 'emergency' caesarean takes place unexpectedly, and there are many reasons why one can take place, for example:

- Labour begins before your scheduled caesarean takes place.
- You or your baby experience a complication during pregnancy or labour and you may be advised to consider a caesarean, for example, a breech presentation.
- Labour stalls or is slow, sometimes known as 'failure to progress' in medical terms. Mum and baby may be fine but a caesarean can be offered.
- You or your baby experience a complication during pregnancy or labour, where your baby needs to be born as quickly as possible. Surgery may take place within 30 minutes of the decision.

The majority of caesareans are not carried out due to immediately urgent and life-threatening circumstances.

What happens before a caesarean birth?

If a caesarean birth is being recommended, then your doctor or midwife should explain why, along with the risks of not having the surgery and the risks of the surgery itself. You should have time to ask any questions you have. You will be asked for your consent and to sign a consent form which says that you understand the risks. You do also have the right to not consent, and to decline a caesarean.

For the surgery itself, you will be asked to change into a hospital gown, and remove all jewellery, make up, nail polish or false nails, dental braces, glasses or contact lenses. Your birth partner can look after your glasses so that you can put them back on after the operation to see your baby.

If you are having a spinal or epidural anaesthetic, you will stay awake, and your birth partner will be able to stay with you during the caesarean. He will need to wear medical scrubs like anyone else who will be in the theatre, to prevent contamination. This will include a facemask, hat and shoe covers, as well as sterile 'scrubs' to cover up their clothing. If you are going to have a general anaesthetic (meaning you will not be awake for the surgery), your birth partner will usually be asked to stay outside the operating theatre.

These are some of the preparations which will be undertaken before the caesarean:

- You will have a blood test for anaemia.
- A drip will be inserted into a vein in your arm for fluids.
- A catheter inserted into your bladder via your urethra.
- A regional anaesthetic that numbs your bottom half, if you are staying awake for the surgery.
- A blood pressure cuff will be put on your upper arm to measure your blood pressure.
- You will have electrodes attached to your chest with tape to monitor your heart rate. You may also have a finger-pulse monitor attached.
- You will have an injection of antibiotics to prevent infection and anti-sickness medicine to prevent vomiting and antacids, in case you need a general anaesthetic.

What happens during a caesarean?

Whether a caesarean is 'elective' or 'emergency', what happens during the surgery itself is likely to remain similar:

- There could be 8–10 people in the operating theatre with you including a surgeon, a midwife, an obstetrician, a theatre nurse, an anaesthetist and probably a paediatrician (doctor specialising in children). There may also be assistants.
- If you will be awake during surgery, a screen will be placed across your chest so you can't see the surgery itself taking

place. You can ask for this to be lowered as your baby is born. If you have had a general anaesthetic, you won't be aware of anything until you wake up.

■ An anaesthetist will check that your painkiller is working properly by asking you. You shouldn't feel any pain at all during the operation, though you may be aware of some sensations like pulling or tugging. As your uterus is opened you may sense fluid whooshing out through the opening, and you may be aware of pressure on your abdomen from where a member of the surgical team pushes down as your baby is pulled out.

■ The time the surgery takes to when your baby is born is relatively quick – usually 5–10 minutes. The stitching after the surgery takes much longer, around 30–45 minutes.

When do I get my baby?

If you are awake and your baby is well, he or she can be handed to you immediately. Your baby can be placed straight onto your chest for skin-to-skin (see page 204) and some women have breastfed their babies while still in theatre! Your midwife will be there to help you. If you don't feel comfortable holding your baby yourself at this point, your birth partner can hold them instead.

If you have had a general anaesthetic, once checked over and assuming all is well, your baby can be given to your birth partner outside the operating theatre.

If your baby needs any help breathing, or has other problems, he or she may need to be taken to the special care baby unit, as with any delivery.

It can feel that with a caesarean birth, that due to all the procedures and people involved, that there isn't much opportunity to have an influence over how things go. However, there are choices and preferences that you can explore together with your partner. Read the Get Together section (see page 171) to find out more about what some of these are.

His

A caesarean section can make you feel like there 'isn't much' that you can do. However, as a birth partner, your role will be just as important in these circumstances, as you are needed to reassure and support your partner.

If your partner is having an epidural, she will be awake during the operation. In most cases you will be welcomed into the surgical theatre to support her during the operation. You will need to wear sterile hospital scrubs to minimise the risk of contamination, which you will be given. There are likely to be 8–10 people in the operating theatre, also in scrubs. There might be sights, sounds and smells that you might find challenging.

If you find yourself feeling anxious during the surgery, try keeping your eyes focused on your partner's face, rather than watch the surgery. Talk about the excitement of very soon meeting your baby. Make use of any of the skills you learnt in antenatal classes for keeping calm and focused, such as breathing practice or other relaxation techniques. It is completely natural that you may be feeling scared, but using these skills will help you to stay as calm as possible, so you can support her.

In Chapter 15 we looked at the two key parts of a birth partners' role: advocate and protector (see page 142), and during a caesarean birth, these two roles are still vital:

Protector role

Your role of protector is so important during a caesarean birth, as the environment of an operating room can be frightening, especially if the caesarean section was unplanned. Supporting your partner to stay as calm as possible will help make the birth experience as positive as possible for you all. It will also minimise how much stress hormone is being passed to your baby during their birth.

Bright lights, lots of people bustling around, preparation for surgery, consent forms and so forth – this can be scary for both of you. As birth partner, it can be very hard to reassure when you are feeling afraid or worried yourself. Try not to place too high expectations on yourself; being there to support and reassure your partner is enough. Holding her hand, stroking her forehead, kissing her cheeks or just talking to her has a massive impact. If you feel able, use a calm, low voice to reassure her that you are staying with her. Support her to use any skills learnt in your antenatal classes for staying calm like breathing practice and relaxation techniques.

Once your baby has been born, assuming your baby does not require additional care, protect the beginning of the bonding experience by keeping the baby close to your partner. Place him or her on your partner's chest for a skin-to-skin cuddle if she feels able/wants to. Your partner might prefer the baby close to her face so she can see them. Those first crucial moments of bonding can be facilitated and protected by you, which is an awesome and significant role.

After the surgery, your partner might experience physical tremors and shakes. This is a normal side-effect following a caesarean, but it can be frightening for your partner. If this happens, reassure her that it is only temporary, stay with her, and ask the midwife for extra blankets.

It is also important to remember that your role as protector doesn't end with the birth. In the first hours, days and weeks following the birth, you can continue to protect your family unit and the developing relationship between your partner and baby. Your partner is likely to need help being passed the baby in the first hours following a caesarean, as she will be unable to move, so help her to do that. In the days and weeks following the birth, it is important to remember that a caesarean section is major abdominal surgery, and recovery while also adjusting to life as a new mum, especially with all the other physical and emotional changes taking place, is a big thing. Protect the space for your partner to be able to recover, whether from too many visitors, or keeping your home vaguely clean and tidy.

When you return to work, talk to your partner about what kind of support she might like you to organise, be it friends, family or hiring a postnatal doula. Make sure your partner is involved so that she can veto or approve any support; it is so important in these early days that she feels comfortable with who will be around, and that she understands you are doing it to support her, not because you don't think she can cope.

Advocate role

A caesarean birth does not automatically mean that you cannot have your preferences fulfilled, and therefore the advocate role remains the same, regardless of the type of birth.

If you have written a birth plan for a vaginal birth but a caesarean birth is needed, it can feel like your birth plan has become irrelevant. However, there are still choices open to you:

- You can choose the relaxation techniques you learned in classes to help keep you both calm.
- You can say what music your partner would like during surgery. An increasing number of hospitals will now play music in the operating room. A 2009 study by the Cochrane Pregnancy and Childbirth Group found that music during caesarean births lowered women's pulse rates and improved their perception of the birth experience. Choosing the music that plays when your child comes into the world is a pretty awesome thing to be able to do!
- You can ask to find out the sex of the baby yourself.
- You can ask to have the screen lowered at the moment of birth, if that is what your partner wants.

- You can ask to have the lights dimmed and to have no talking at the moment of birth.
- You can ask for your partner to have skin-to-skin contact with your partner straight after birth, keeping mum and baby together during the stitching.

Some of these preferences may not be possible if there is a problem, as any reasonable person knows, but in the event that all goes smoothly, they are an important part of the birth experience that you can advocate for.

When you are not able to be at a caesarean birth

Sometimes caesarean births are done under general anaesthetic, which means your partner is not awake during the surgery and birth and you are unlikely to be allowed in the room. This can be an extraordinarily difficult position to be in, especially if the caesarean is decided on in an emergency and you are left not knowing what is happening while your partner is rushed out to surgery. It is not uncommon to feel a mix of emotions from anger to grief, or to experience shaking or crying from the rush of adrenalin you may experience.

If this situation should occur, a midwife should come and talk to you to explain what is happening. He or she will do this after your partner is ready in theatre, as the wellbeing and safety of her and your baby will take priority. While this can be very hard on you, you can take some comfort in the fact that the reason they have not come to talk to you yet is because everyone is focused on your partner and baby.

Any coping tools you have learnt in your antenatal preparation are really useful to use while your partner is in surgery; use them to help you keep calm until there is more news. Someone will tell you when your baby has been born, and how your partner and baby are doing. If all is well with your baby, he or she may even be brought out to you, and this is something you can specifically request.

Looking after your baby until you are reunited with your partner isn't something to be too anxious about; all that your baby will really want and need in those first minutes are lots of cuddles. Talk to your baby, cuddle and rock him or her. If you wish to have skin-to-skin contact with your baby you can do his too. Find a chair, open or take off your top, and put your naked baby against your chest, covered with a blanket to keep them warm. Ask your midwife for support to do this if you need, as she is there to support you all as a family unit. If mum had wanted skin-to-skin after birth as part of your original birth plan, this can be a nice way of making sure baby still gets this, even if it isn't with her yet.

Don't rush to get baby dressed; you can keep them covered with a blanket, and it can be nice when mum awakes for her to see her baby as he or she first came into the world, and to have the option of some skin-to-skin time too. Your partner may feel a lot of control was taken away from her during the birth, so it is important that she feels a part of the choices which now happen after birth, including simple things like choosing baby's first outfit.

Get Together

If you are planning an elective caesarean, we would highly suggest working together to create a caesarean birth plan. A caesarean birth experience does not have to be a traumatic experience, and there are choices you can explore and discuss.

It cannot be ignored that a caesarean section is surgery, and sometimes due to this, they can become more process-focused than family-centred. But, your caesarean is your birth, and needs to be treated as one. While not every preference on your list might be able to be facilitated, it is only by asking that you are likely to get any of them!

So here are some things to think about when you're deciding what kind of caesarean birth experience you would like:

When to have the caesarean

When would you like your caesarean birth to be? While most are scheduled for 37–38 weeks, if you wish, you can express an alternative preference. You could request waiting until as close to 'due date' as possible, so that your baby has had more time to finish developing. Bear in mind that due dates can be inaccurate, so 38 weeks could actually be earlier or later in terms of your baby's development. You could request that you would like to wait until your body starts very early labour, so you know your baby has given the signal that she or he is now ready to be born.

Pain relief

You will require pain relief for a caesarean birth, and there should be the opportunity to discuss your choices with an anaesthetist. Broadly, your choices are:

- A regional anaesthetic, which numbs the abdomen and enables you to stay awake for the birth. This is likely to be administered as a one-off injection called a spinal, but an epidural can also be used. If you have a regional anaesthetic, the birth partner should be able to be present from the beginning to the end of the caesarean.
- A general anaesthetic, which means being asleep for the birth. This has more risks for mum and baby and is usually only used when a situation is urgent, as it can be administered much more quickly. Sometimes, there are other circumstances which might make this a preferential choice for

birth, so discuss it with your doctor. If your caesarean is carried out under general anaesthetic, the obstetrician may not allow your partner into the operating theatre. Ask if your partner can be just outside the theatre door so he can hold your baby as soon as possible, if that's important to you.

Birth environment

There will be aspects of the birth environment that you may not be able to change, but there will be plenty that you can express a preference about, to help create a unique and individual birth experience for you:

- Music playing in the background or a specific piece of music being played as your baby is born?
- A running commentary from the theatre staff about what is happening, so you can feel more involved in the birth progress?
- Silence at the moment baby is lifted out, so the first voice your baby hears is yours?
- The lights to be dimmed a little as baby is lifted out, to make the transition into the world less of a shock to the system?
- The screen to be lowered so you can see your baby being born?
- Someone to take photos or video of the birth?

Parenting preferences

As with a vaginal birth, your birth plan doesn't stop at the birth of your baby, and there are many choices you can make for the first moments after birth (see page 199):

- Whether you wish to discover the sex of your baby for yourselves, or to be told by the medical team?

- Whether either of you want to have skin-to-skin with your baby?
- Whether you want to try breastfeeding your baby as soon as you can?
- Whether you would like the medical team to facilitate delayed cord clamping (see page 206)?
- Whether you would like to see or keep the placenta (see page 207)?
- What would you would like your baby's cord clamped with?

A caesarean birth is still always a birth, so spend some time together discussing what preferences you have, to make it a positive birth experience for you all.

CHAPTER 18

Vaginal birth after caesarean

A vaginal birth after a caesarean is also known as a VBAC (pronounced 'vee back'). It simply means giving birth to your baby vaginally when you've had a previous baby by caesarean section.

Hers

If you have previously given birth by caesarean, you will be offered the option of an elective caesarean section. This doesn't mean that having a vaginal birth is not possible or is 'dangerous' and evidence actually shows that a VBAC is safer for mother and baby than elective caesarean.

If you have had a caesarean birth previously, when you had hoped for a vaginal birth, you may have a strong desire to experience a vaginal birth. There are many positives to having a VBAC, including:

- You avoid the risks associated with surgery and anaesthetic that come with major abdominal surgery.

- Less risk of infection.
- Shorter time spent in hospital.
- Increased likelihood of immediate contact with your baby.
- A lower risk of your baby developing breathing problems.
- A reduced recovery time, which with other children at home is important.
- A lower risk of complications in future pregnancies. The risk of some complications, such as hysterectomy or placental problems, rises with every caesarean a woman has. This means that, when working out the balance of risks and benefits, you should take into account whether you hope to have more children after this current pregnancy.

However, some women are apprehensive about the idea of a VBAC, especially if there has been a previous difficult birth experience. It is not uncommon to feel that you would rather plan a repeat caesarean, than have the worry that an attempt at vaginal birth would end in caesarean anyway. The chances of a successful vaginal birth vary according to various factors, such as the reasons for your past caesarean, and the number of past caesareans you have had. It is worth knowing that most women who choose a VBAC do have a vaginal birth. There is a variance between hospitals, but most show VBAC rates of over 70 per cent.

Some women are concerned about the risk of uterine rupture (the uterine scar from an earlier caesarean not coping with labour and breaking open). There is an increased risk of this during VBAC, compared with a woman who has not had a caesarean before, but it is still a very low risk. It is also important to understand that some women are at higher risk of uterine rupture than others; not all VBAC attempts are equally safe. Evidence shows that induction, for example, increases the likelihood. Being aware of this is crucial to inform your decision-making.

If you want to have a VBAC there are ways you can maximise your chances of achieving a vaginal birth. These are not unique to VBAC; they are actually exactly the same actions as for any woman wanting to maximise her opportunity for a vaginal birth, and include:

- Choose a place of birth where you feel safe and comfortable.
- Choose a health care team who support your desire to have a vaginal birth.
- Have a clear birth plan and discuss this with your midwife/consultant in advance.
- Allow your body to start labour naturally.
- Allow your body to progress labour in its own time, with no time limits, and don't opt for being induced, including having your waters broken or a syntocinon drip.
- Stay at home for as long as you feel comfortable and confident.
- Request intermittent fetal monitoring rather than continuous monitoring.
- Stay mobile and relaxed – have tools to help you do this such as a birth ball, breathing practice and relaxation techniques.

When planning a VBAC it is important to consider who your birth partner is and how they feel about your preferences; their support is a crucial factor in the likelihood you will achieve your goal. Make time to discuss how he feels about your desire for a vaginal birth, and why he feels that way. If he was present at a previous birth and witnessed any trauma, he may still be affected. This can lead him to feel a certain way about vaginal birth and think that a caesarean is safer.

It is important for you to discuss your wishes with him, as your birth partner is a crucial part of your birth plan. Can he be an advocate if you are put under pressure to make a choice that is not in line with your preferences?

His

There are a lot of resources, information and support for VBAC mums. But what about VBAC dads?

If you were present at a birth that didn't go to plan, and resulted in an emergency caesarean, you may have strong feelings about the idea of a VBAC. Many men (though not all) feel that it is safer for their partner to plan to have a subsequent caesarean rather than a vaginal birth. The evidence suggests that a VBAC is safer in most cases than a repeat caesarean, so why is it that so many men feel this way?

What is hard for some guys to admit is that we might have our own issues from a previous birth. If a previous hoped-for vaginal birth became an emergency caesarean, we may be carrying memories of a frightening time and have our own trauma that we have not yet worked through. As partners we want to be sure that our partner and baby will be okay. If we have witnessed a vaginal birth 'go wrong', it is understandable that thinking that going straight for a caesarean this time is the better option.

You might not be sure how to support your partner through a vaginal birth. You might feel unequipped to advocate her wishes if she feels under pressure from friends, family or medical professionals to have another caesarean.

It is important to acknowledge how your personal feelings and fears do affect your partner's choices, and the likelihood of achieving the birth they want. Many women do not feel that VBAC is an option for them, not because they don't want one, but because their partner isn't keen on the idea. It's important to recognise how potentially significant your influence is on your partner's decision-making. She may feel she cannot pursue VBAC without feeling that you are 100 per cent behind her.

This matters, because for women, how their baby arrives into the world can be incredibly important. The relationship between a mother and child is strongly linked to the birth, and it is an emotional decision for most women. Vaginal birth is something that women's bodies are designed to do, and it is a unique, primal act that many women feel the need to experience. However, this desire does not mean 'at any cost', and most women who want a VBAC just want support for a vaginal birth as long as she and baby are fine.

Is a repeat caesarean safer and easier?

A caesarean is a fairly safe surgery, but it is still major abdominal surgery. It therefore carries with it significant risks, including infection. The recovery can be more intense and limiting than a vaginal birth, which can be made more difficult if there are other children to care for.

Something which men (and women) have often unspoken worry about is the risk of maternal mortality; the possibility of mum dying during birth. It is this fear that leads many to choose the seemingly 'safer' option of a caesarean. However, this is a great example of where assumption and evidence are contradictory. For example, one study in the Netherlands between 1983 and 1992 found that the death rate from caesareans was seven times that from vaginal birth. Having a vaginal birth after a caesarean does carry with it an increased risk of a uterine rupture, but it is a very small increased risk (the risk is under 1 per cent). While any complications depend on the individual circumstances and medical background of mum, understanding that a caesarean is not automatically the safest option is important.

A VBAC is much easier to achieve with the wholehearted support of a partner and birth partner. If you want to support your partner to have a VBAC, but feel that you lack the skills or confidence, look into hiring a doula (see page 147) to give you and your partner the support you need. If you both wish for you to be the VBAC birth partner, get involved in learning skills to support your partner with labour from as early in pregnancy as possible. Support your partner to explore the choices open to you both. Act as your partner's advocate towards the end of the pregnancy. VBAC is a shared experience and has shared responsibility – you matter!

Get Together

I f you wish to have a VBAC, make time to discuss how you both feel about it, and all the options open to you. Many parents worry that their choices will be limited – this is not the case, you still have a large number of choices open to you, but some you may have more support for than others. They still, however, remain your choices.

It is important that you can work together, or bring in another birth partner who can support you if necessary. Being able to respect preferences can be a crucial part of making a VBAC a reality.

The support you receive for your wish to have a VBAC will vary according to what hospital you are at, the views of the consultant or midwife responsible for your care, and your individual circumstances. If you wish to have a VBAC but are not feeling support for your decision, you have choices. You can:

- Follow the advice of not having a VBAC, whether you feel this is the best thing for you, or not.
- Ask to be referred to a different obstetrician, who may be more supportive.
- Make contact with the supervisor of midwives to discuss your preferences and seek support.

- Stay with your current health care team, but decline their advice and choose a vaginal birth. Under NICE (see page 46) guidance, they should support your right to make an informed decision.

Can we have a VBAC at home?

Having your baby in a non-medicalised environment greatly increases the likelihood of having a non-medicalised birth, so many families who wish to achieve a VBAC take this into account to increase their chances.

If you had a previous bad experience in hospital, or you have negative associations with hospital for any reason, giving birth at home might also be important to you.

The risk of a serious problem occurring in labour are not massively increased just because you have had a previous caesarean. However, it can be helpful to take into account how long a transfer to hospital would take if you did need one, as there are always some risks. The advice for women with a uterine scar is to be within 30 minutes of emergency medical assistance.

You have the right, even if you have had a previous caesarean, to choose to stay at home to give birth. You can contact the supervisor of midwives to discuss your plan to birth at home and to seek support. You could also choose to hire an independent midwife, if you feel you are not getting the support you need.

What are the options for monitoring during a VBAC?

NICE guidelines say that continuous foetal monitoring should be offered to women having a VBAC. However, this is 'offered' not 'required', and monitoring always, ultimately, remains your choice and requires your consent.

It is interesting to note that there is no reliable evidence to show that continuous monitoring makes VBAC safer.

A Cochrane review (see page 169) found that continuous monitoring is not more effective at picking up distress in babies than intermittent monitoring. In addition, the review found continuous monitoring does not reduce the number of babies that die, and makes no difference to the long-term health of babies born.

The Cochrane review, did however, clearly show that continuous monitoring increases the number of unnecessary caesareans carried out, which means that it can reduce the likelihood of a VBAC. Your choices for monitoring during a VBAC include:

- No monitoring at all.
- Intermittent monitoring with a sonic aid or similar hand-held device.
- Continuous monitoring with a wireless monitor to enable staying mobile.
- Continuous monitoring.
- A combination of the above as you prefer.

Should I have an induction?

Research suggests that women whose labours are induced or augmented are at increased risk of uterine rupture following a caesarean. If you decline induction, your risk of uterine rupture is therefore reduced.

You can choose to decline an induction for a VBAC as you can during any vaginal birth. It is important to be aware of the implications if you do so, as there might be other choices that you will need to make, which may be against the usual protocols of your care provider. For example, waiting for labour to start of its own accord will mean you may wish to consider how long you are happy to wait, whether it is 40 weeks, 42 weeks or beyond this. If you wait until things happen naturally, you should be offered regular monitoring to check how baby is doing.

Declining augmentation, means that during labour, you wait for things to progress at their own pace, or choose a caesarean. Opting for a caesarean once labour has begun, will mean it will be classed as an emergency caesarean.

Can I have a VBAC water birth?

Yes, although it may vary as to how supportive of your preference your care providers are. If birthing in a hospital, gain support for labouring in water with your consultant, and have him or her make a supporting statement on your notes. If you cannot gain support from the hospital to use their birth pool, you may wish to consider the option of hiring one to use at home, and discuss your preference with the supervisor of midwives.

CHAPTER 19

Induction of labour

Did you know that 25–32 per cent of labours are induced, and many more involve an augmentation? Induction and augmentation can make a big difference to your birth experience, so understanding more about these interventions, and knowing that you have choices about whether to have them or not, is really important.

Hers

Induction of labour basically means kick-starting labour rather than letting it start of its own accord. Augmentation of labour means using a medical intervention to help labour along, with the aim that it progresses more quickly.

Induction and augmentation will be offered when medical professionals believe it is safer for mum and baby to birth earlier or more quickly. However, induction can also be offered for reasons which are a bit less clear. For example, when labour has not started by itself, or soon after the due date, even if everything else looks good with mum and baby in the antenatal checks. Induction may also be offered if there is a belief that your baby may be 'big', which could be true, although scans are notoriously inaccurate for predicting baby's weight, and it is common for babies who are predicted to be 'big', to be born at a very average size.

NICE guidance acknowledges that there is an increased likelihood of requiring pain relief and an assisted delivery with induction, and recommends that parents are told this in discussions about induction. In first-time parents, there is also evidence that suggest a correlation between induction and caesarean section. Induction can have an impact not only on your birth this time, but also on subsequent births, as women who have a caesarean with their first baby, are more likely to have them with subsequent pregnancies.

Choosing whether or not to be induced is often not an easy decision; there are benefits and risks to consider on both sides. You need to work out what risks you are both prepared to take, what benefits matter to you, if there are measures you can use to minimise any risks, and ultimately, doing what you feel is right in your circumstances. We all want to take the safest or risk-free option for our family, but the reality is that there is always a risk (and potential benefit) with every choice.

Let's consider one example: if you are offered induction because you have reached 41 weeks of pregnancy, then you should have the risks of induction explained to you, as well as the risks attached to prolonging a pregnancy past 42 weeks.

If you are offered induction for a medical reason, such as pre-eclampsia, again the medical professionals should explain to you both the risks of induction, but also the risks with continuing the pregnancy.

If you are offered induction, your choices include:

- Accepting medical induction.
- Declining medical induction.
- Requesting increased monitoring.
- Trying natural means of induction (see page 195).

It is very usual for women to feel fed up with being pregnant near the end of pregnancy. You might be tired, not sleeping well, feel uncomfortable, and might face a host of symptoms. You might feel ready to meet your baby. I have known women ask if they can have a stretch and sweep earlier than 40 weeks, not for any medical reason, but just because they want their baby to be here. I always feel that women at the end of their pregnancy are in a more vulnerable place, as we like the idea of meeting baby soon, so the idea of induction can appeal, even if previously we have felt that it was not something we wanted. A couple of things to bear in mind here:

- It is okay to change your mind. Maybe you didn't want to be induced, but now you do. This is okay. Make sure you make your decision an informed and individual one. Be clear about what you want and don't want, and what you can do to support the process.
- You can say 'no', 'not yet' or 'yes' later on. Just because you decide not to be induced today, doesn't mean that you can't make a different decision tomorrow. Take it one day at a time, and one decision at a time.
- Patience can be difficult. Waiting for labour to start is the supreme test of the ability to be patient, and some of us cope better with that than others. For some people it is all part of the great surprise, while others find the lack of certainty makes them anxious. This is all understandable. Even with induction however, you still don't know when your baby will arrive.
- One word of caution: if your body is not ready to birth, induction can be a long process; it is not unusual for it to take a few days. You are likely to be in hospital for all this time, and your partner might not able to stay with you overnight, if that is the hospital policy. One of the most common things that women report back, is being shocked at how long their induction took.

It can be possible to get an idea of how the induction might go before it begins. Your care team use the Bishop's Score to assess what is happening in your body, and whether it is 'favourable' to induction. Being favourable means that your body has already started making changes as it has prepares for labour to begin. You can ask to know what the result of the Bishop's Score is, to help make your decision. Some people feel that if their body has not started making preparations, then the induction is less likely to work and so they want to delay it, or avoid it altogether (either waiting for labour to happen of its own accord, or conversely, requesting a caesarean instead of the induction).

If your body if is ready to go into labour anyway, then induction can be helpful as a quick nudge to get things underway. Consider though, if your body is ready to go into labour anyway, it will probably happen naturally within a couple of days.

There is a lot to think about, but whatever you choose, it is completely your choice. This means that if your midwife says, 'you are 40 weeks on your next appointment, so I will do a stretch and sweep', you can say 'no', 'not yet' as well as 'okay'. You can also ask for more information or say that you will think about it and decide later. If you are at 41 weeks of pregnancy and are told: 'I will book you in this week for a hospital induction', you can still say 'no', 'not yet' as well as 'okay'. You can also still ask for more information, or say you will think about it and make your choice later.

A key part of how we work with parents is never telling or advising someone what they should do, but we do think it is important that parents understand that they do always have a choice. We have worked with couples who came to us for support to prepare for second or third babies, who tell us that for their first birth they: 'had to be induced, there was no choice.' There is always a choice, and it is important you know this so that you can be a part of that decision-making.

If you decide to have an induction, be involved in weighing up the risks and benefits. Then if things don't go to plan, you know that you made your choice for all the right reasons despite it not quite working out as hoped. This is much better than feeling like it was something done to you which you had no power over, or that there were other options you didn't know about. Feeling powerless and out of control is most often a negative experience. Feeling in control and empowered, even if things don't go to plan, is more likely to be a positive experience.

Planning for a positive induction

An induction is still part of your birth plan, so you need to say what you want and don't want, rather than feeling like you have no choices or preferences.

Induction can take a while to get going, so make sure you have plenty to keep you occupied. Once labour is starting, try anything you think will help; go for a walk, go outdoors, go and get a snack from the hospital shop, look at your scan picture or photos of your other children. Put on some special music and use your birth anchors to make your space yours, so you feel safe enough to allow labour to progress.

During induction, it is likely that you will be asked if you want to be monitored. This is to check how your baby is coping with the intervention, and the labour that arises from it. There is a risk, with all methods of induction, of baby becoming distressed, which is why it is part of the routine process to periodically check on them. You may be asked to lie on the bed for monitoring, but you can choose to remain in a more mobile position such as standing, kneeling, all-fours or sitting on a birth ball. Tell your midwife what you are doing to be comfortable: don't ask for permission, just ask for his or her support to work with what you need. Ask if the hospital has wireless monitoring, which means you can even continue to walk around a room or get in a bath! Even if you need to be attached to a drip, it is still possible to remain in a more active position.

Make sure you support your body to work as efficiently as possible, so drink plenty of fluids, eat nutritious snacks, and wee regularly (see page 151).

During an induction, using any skills you learnt in antenatal classes to keep calm and relaxed is really important. With all the nervous energy of going in for an induction, plus the fact that your body doesn't know it is time for labour, you need to do everything you can to encourage the oxytocin (see page 130) to flow, while minimising the flow of adrenalin (see page 130).

Be aware that some hospitals have a policy of sending fathers home at night if labour hasn't kicked in or is still only in the early stages. Have a plan with your partner for what you will do if this happens.

If a medical intervention is suggested and you are not sure about it, ask your partner to use the BRAIN tool (see page 191) with the medical professionals, to help you understand what is being offered and why. Ask for time alone with your partner to discuss it, before making a decision. If you are fine and your baby is fine, there may be no need to have further interventions.

If the induction is difficult, long, or you are struggling, you can always say that you want the treatment to stop and you do not consent to any further induction interventions. Ask for a caesarean if that feels right for you. At the end of the day, there is nothing wrong with this as a choice if it will give you a more positive birth experience and if it feels right for you and your baby.

His

A crucial part of your advocate role is helping to weigh up options when your partner is offered a choice just before or during birth. This is especially important when an induction is being suggested.

The very first thing to do in this situation, is to ask the medical professionals if it is an emergency, and whether there is time to talk the suggested intervention through. Assuming there is time (and 99 per cent of the time, there will be) then you can use the 'BRAIN' method to work things out logically. In birth, there can be a lot of emotion (as it is such an important time) so having a way of looking at the facts is helpful. You both need to consider:

B – What are the **BENEFITS** to the offered intervention? How will it help your partner, your child and you as a family?

R – What are the **RISKS**? Consider all the risks and, crucially, how likely they are to happen? There is a big difference between a 50 per cent risk and a 0.01 per cent risk! If you have been told your risk will double, ask, 'double from what to what?' Doubling from 30 per cent to 60 per cent is one thing, but if it is doubling from 0.1 per cent to 0.2 per cent this is another. How do you both feel about the relative risk? What are the risks to our partner, to our baby and also are there any risks associated to our family later on? Can going forward on one course of action now, restrict our choices in other ways later on?

A – Now you understand what the benefits and risks are, ask about any **ALTERNATIVES**. What other choices are open to you? Remember, there is never only one choice.

I – What does **INTUITION** tell you? Sometimes you both might need some time, be it ten minutes or an hour, to sit and really tune in to what you feel is right for you. Ask your partner what her intuition is saying to her. What feels like the right course of action?

N – Finally, you always have the choice to do **NOTHING**. Ask the question: so what if we do nothing for the moment? Can we just have a little more time?

As with any tool, the more you can practise this before the day you need to use it, the more confident you will be with it. You could use it as you consider the different options as you write your birth plan together (see page 111). Use it to consider options such as where to give birth, pain relief, after baby has been born, and so on.

What is my role if we choose to be induced?

Your role stays the same, albeit with a few little tweaks! An induction is still part of your birth experience, so your role of advocate is crucial as it would be with any birth. Support your partner to be heard in terms of what is important to her.

Induction can be a bit of a slow process to begin, so be prepared for how to fill the time. Make sure that you are able to keep mum distracted with magazines, books or whatever it is which she enjoys to pass the time while she waits. She may be too nervous or excited to focus on something, so be aware and if necessary be ready to just talk to her, go for a walk or bring her a little treat from the hospital shop. Once labour is starting, go into your protector role and try and cultivate a positive environment for birthing. Put on the music you have chosen for labour, get your partner into comfortable clothing or on a birth ball.

If you partner is monitored during induction, support her if she requests that she would like to be in a more upright or mobile position. Women are often requested to lie on the bed for monitoring, to make it easier to keep the straps in the right place, but it is not impossible to also monitor baby in other positions. As we looked at in Chapter 14, lying down comes with its own risks. If your baby needs to be monitored support your partner, advocate for whatever position she is comfortable in – being on a ball, standing up, on all fours… Ask if they have wireless monitoring which means she really can be mobile.

Support your partner by making sure that she is drinking enough (this is vital to ensure her uterine muscles work effectively). Remember the bendy straws that you packed in your birth bag. Remind her to go to the toilet, once an hour as a general guide. An empty bladder gives the baby more space to move down.

Support your partner to use any skills you learnt in antenatal classes to keep calm and relaxed; these can be so important during an induction when there can be a lot of anticipatory adrenalin.

Many hospitals have a policy of not allowing fathers to stay overnight if labour is not yet in full flow. This can mean leaving your partner on an antenatal ward in the early stages of labour. Consider what you will do in this circumstance. You need to be rested in order to be able to support her when labour does get doing, but you will also want to be contactable and able to return quickly if you are suddenly needed. Discuss with your partner how she feels about the possibility of you leaving, and what she can do to manage in your absence. Find out what the hospital policy is on this, and if there is a way of overcoming it. Do they have a private room which you can pay to use, for example?

Get Together

Induction is a common intervention, but because it happens before labour begins, often parents miss it off their birth plan. Given that one-in-four labours are induced in the UK, and induction will usually massively impact on how the birth unfolds and some of the choices available to you both, it is important to see it as part of your birth plan, and to think in advance about how you feel about it.

Use the following as a starting point to discuss how you feel about induction for dates, as you are likely to be offered a sweep if you reach 40 weeks, and a hospital induction if you reach 41 weeks. However, also revisit this information and discussion if you are offered induction for a specific reason. Obviously you can only weigh up induction versus waiting once you know what the specific reason for induction being recommended is.

What are the options if we are offered induction?
Option 1: To say no.

You can always say no. Induction is your choice. NICE guidelines state: 'If a woman chooses not to have induction of labour, her decision should be respected. Healthcare professionals should discuss the woman's care with her from then on.'

If you do decline the induction of labour, you should be offered regular monitoring to check how your baby is, and if there are any concerns at all, professionals can let you know so you can reassess your decision to wait.

It is also helpful to think about the fact that you can say no, meaning not today. Saying no today doesn't mean you can't change your mind and say yes tomorrow.

Option 2. Try natural methods of induction first

If you want to get things moving but don't want to use medi-calised means, you could try natural methods to kick start things. Whether these are 'old wives tales' or there is something more to them is up for debate, but it is a choice for parents-to-be. You might want to try:

- **Sex**. Not always highest priority on the list when you are heavily pregnant, as it can be tricky, but making love releases the labour hormone oxytocin (see page 130). Also, semen contains prostaglandins which help soften the cervix.

- **Hugs**. If sex isn't on the agenda, cuddles and hugs have a similar oxytocin-boosting effect.

- **Eat some spicy food**. It is thought that the spices stimulate the bowel, which gets things moving. It is not proven to be effective, but is well worth a try if you like spicy food.

- **Nipple stimulation**. Again this can stimulate the hormone oxytocin.

- **Walking**. Harnessing gravity to encourage the baby to drop further, stimulating the release of oxytocin.

- **Acupressure or acupuncture**. Many testify to this getting labour going, and it is usually a nice relaxing method to try, too.

One small word of warning with all of these options, is that, no matter how natural this all is, it is still an attempted intervention/induction. This means that some of these methods may have side-effects, such as an upset tummy from the spicy food, or labour beginning very strongly from an acupressure treatment.

Option 3. Choose medical induction

If you choose a medical induction, there are several methods which can be used. This will usually be determined following monitoring, a vaginal examination and using the 'Bishop's Score' (see page 188).

The vaginal examination is to determine how 'favourable' the cervix is, whether your body has started making progress in terms of preparation for labour. If your cervix is deemed 'favourable' it means that induction is more likely to be successful. However, if the check shows the cervix is unfavourable, then induction is less likely to work, which is a pretty common sense way of looking at it!

The method of induction offered could be:

- **A sweep**. Normally carried out by a midwife. Similar to a vaginal examination, the midwife will insert her fingers into your vagina, stretching the cervix and sweeping her fingers across the membrane. Sometimes this can stimulate contractions within the next day or so. However, a sweep may not have any effect. Risks which are not common, but to bear in mind include accidentally breaking the waters, and as with any vaginal examination, there is always a risk of introduction of infection.

- **Pessary, tablet or gel**: These products contain prostaglandin, a hormone that can help soften the cervix. The product is inserted into the vagina. Risks of this method can include uterine hyper-stimulation, which means contractions last longer and come more frequently than should be safely expected. Uterine hyper-stimulation can lead to uterine rupture, foetal distress and other associated complications.

- **Artificial rupture of the membranes**: This means artificially breaking the bag of waters around your baby. The midwife inserts an instrument into the vagina and through the cervix to rupture the waters. The aim is to remove the cushion of water between your baby and cervix, to put more pressure on the cervix with the aim of increasing the pace of labour.

Whether evidence supports this practice is a subject up for debate. One review of the studies reported that it did not make the first stage of labour go any quicker, while there was a possible link to an increase in caesarean section. Risks include increase in the intensity of contractions felt by mum and foetal distress.

- **Syntocinon**: This is an artificial form of oxytocin, the hormone that stimulates labour. It is normally administered through an IV drip in the hand. Syntocinon brings on contractions, which can be very strong. Guidance under NICE states that if you are offered syntocinon, you should also be told that it is more likely that you will need pain relief during labour. Risks include uterine hyperstimulation and the associated risks (see above), as well as side effects such as nausea, headaches, fall in blood pressure and heart problems.

How will induction affect our birth preferences?

Consider how you feel about the following potential knock-on effects from an induction:

- Dad may need to leave overnight, even if mum is in early labour.
- There may be restrictions on some birthing choices, for example, hospital policy may prohibit you from using a birthing pool or to be on a midwife-led unit.
- A full induction will need to take place in hospital, so you wouldn't be able to give birth at home.
- You are more likely to need pain relief during labour.
- You are more likely to have an assisted birth.

CHAPTER 20

Baby's arrival

Suddenly your baby is here. We can have expectations of those first moments which we may not even be aware we have created; how we expect it to look, what we expect will happen, how we expect to feel. Our experience may completely blow those expectations out of the water, in ways which might be more wonderful than we imagined, or conversely, in ways we had not imagined at all.

Hers

When your baby arrives you may immediately feel an overwhelming sense of love towards him or her. You might feel a strong bond, not wanting to put your baby down and wanting to keep him or her close to you. If you feel this way, keep your baby close; you don't have to pass them around or put them down. This is your baby and you can hold him or her as much as you wish.

The hour after birth is also known as the 'golden hour'. In an undisturbed labour, oxytocin levels continue to build up and up, so that at the time baby is born, oxytocin is at an all-time high, ready to support bonding between mother and the baby. This is a very precious time. To support this amazing bonding opportunity, you need to be kept warm and comfortable with your baby. Lying or sitting skin to-skin with your baby also supports the bonding, as newborn babies bond through touch and smell. Your room should be kept quiet and dark to imitate a womb-like state, which makes it easier for the baby to focus on getting to know its mum, without potential distraction from bright lights, loud noises or other distractions.

However, many women (and men) don't feel these things. It is not unusual to not feel an overwhelming sense of love or an immediate bond. There is nothing wrong with you, or your baby, if this is your experience. Labour and birth can leave you feeling exhausted and this can impact on your feelings at this time. If you have had a birth with interventions, this can impact on your hormone production at birth. If you feel unable to hold your baby after birth, this can also impact on your feelings. Your baby may have been born with a health problem, which may make parents feel worried or distressed. Being surprised or disappointed about your baby's gender can affect the way you bond with your baby at first. Parents who have twins may find bonding with both babies a challenge at first, and this can be made more challenging if one baby needs to be cared for in the neonatal unit (NNU) while the other baby stays with mum on the postnatal ward.

In short, how you feel after your birth can be affected by a whole range of factors, and is one of the secrets that many people don't talk about. The expectation is that you are meant to fall head-over-heels in love with your baby the second he or she is born, and if this doesn't happen immediately, people worry that something is wrong with them. There isn't.

While Mother Nature sets the conditions for bonding to be optimal at birth (which makes sense for mammals birthing in the wild; if they don't bond with their offspring immediately, they would be in danger), it is not a case that if you don't bond in those first couple of hours that you won't. Bonding is optimal in those first couple of hours, there are still plenty of other opportunities to bond in the following hours, days and weeks.

An unexpected appearance

If you haven't seen a newborn baby before, you may be shocked if your baby doesn't look like the 'perfect' images we are shown on TV shows and magazine covers (which are often not newborns!)

When you see your newborn baby for the first time, you may notice:

- Your baby's head may look misshapen and 'cone-shaped'. This is the result of the normal moulding that happens as the baby descends through the pelvis and birth canal. Within a day or two it settles into a rounder shape.
- You may notice a pulsating spot on top of the baby's head, known the 'soft spot' or 'fontanelle'. This is your baby's skull bones have not yet come together, which is again, normal to help ease their birth.
- Your baby's skin may be covered in vernix, a waxy white substance, and this is more common in babies who arrive a little earlier. There is no reason to wash it off as the skin naturally absorbs it.
- Baby's eyes may appear cross-eyed. This is normal. At birth a baby's eyes and eye muscles are learning to function in response to light and movement. As the weeks pass, the eye muscles get stronger and more symmetrical in their movements.
- A baby boy's scrotum may look relatively large compared with the rest of him; sometimes baby boys may also have swollen breast tissue. Baby girls often have slightly swollen labia and breast tissue, and sometimes even have a little 'period'. These are the normal effects of the pregnancy hormones and won't last.

- Baby's hands and feet may feel cold or look slightly blue while the body temperature and circulation systems develop.
- Baby's legs may look bowed. This is purely as an adaptation to the cramped conditions of the uterus. As the muscles strengthen and lengthen, the legs will slowly stretch out over the weeks.
- About 1-in-3 babies have a birthmark, with twice as many girls than boys having one. Most don't hurt the baby, cause health problems or need any treatment.

His

C ongratulations! Your baby is here. Those first moments can feel overwhelming as suddenly it is all very real – you are a dad and you have a baby! You might be grinning from ear-to-ear, you might have some emotional tears, or you might feel a kind of disbelief; all these feelings are normal.

As birth partner, while all of this is quite amazing, your role is not quite over yet. You still need to make sure that the birth preferences you made for after the birth are being followed or discussed. Make sure the midwives know your preference for cord clamping and the third stage, and check with mum she is still happy with her choice. If you are planning a natural third stage (see page 205), protecting the environment to keep the oxytocin flowing is important. Your partner needs to birth the placenta and to be checked for any tears which might need repair. Hold your partner's hand and help her to keep your baby close during this time.

Try to take a few photos of those first moments, and ask your midwife to take your first photograph all together as a family.

Don't be in a rush to leave, to spread the news or get some food. A good rule of thumb is to hang around until your partner is dressed in some clean pyjamas and has a cup of tea to hand and tells you that she feels ok to be left alone!

You can request for any routine procedures to wait until after the 'golden hour' has finished, so in this time just be together getting to know your baby. This is a once-in-a-lifetime opportunity, so enjoy those first moments as a family. Welcome your newborn, take time to hold him or her, and tell your partner how proud of her you are.

Once it is time to make an announcement, make sure you have all the info to hand which you want to share. Date of birth, time of birth, weight, and name are the information that people will be keen to hear! In the world of social media, news travels very quickly, so if you are only telling a few people and you wish to make 'proper' announcement later in your own time, make this clear to them. You might want to limit how many people you tell to try and minimise accidental sharing of the news.

Get Together

Within the first few seconds of your baby's birth, you will already be making parenting choices! It is important to know what your choices are, so that you can make an informed decision. Regardless of what kind of birth you had, you will be able to have some of your preferences followed. So what are those choices open to you, and what are the implications? Here they are for you to discuss:

How soon after birth do you want routine interventions?
In some maternity settings it is still common practice to focus on the medical side of a newborn's health, which can inhibit

your bonding time together. Obviously, some babies will need medical attention after birth, but in the majority of cases they do not, and the opportunity to enhance this important time between parents and baby is missed for no pressing reason.

Routine procedures such as weighing the baby, physical examinations, giving vitamin K (see page 208) and so forth can wait, if you choose. You can request for these things to be done after the first hour (the 'golden' hour), and be left alone to just enjoy your baby. You are also entitled to decline anything you do not wish your baby to have.

What kind of environment after birth do you want?

If you imagine birth from your baby's point of view, it is rather amazing to think of what a major change they experience. Your baby has only known the warm, confined, dark, muffled environment of the womb. He or she had constant contact with their mum, with her voice and heartbeat always present. Then, suddenly, they arrive into a cold, loud, bright world, the safety of the uterus gone. What a shock to the system! How can we support our baby to not have such a shock? Consider the environment that he or she is born into, and what we do to that environment in the first few minutes and hours. Aim to keep your room/s quiet, dark, warm and private. This all helps with a gentler transition and bonding, and the flow of oxytocin.

Skin-to-skin contact

When your baby is born, your first choice is where do you want them to go? Newborn babies bond through touch and smell, which is one of the reasons midwives will encourage skin-to-skin contact. This simply means placing a newborn baby naked on to mum's chest, immediately after birth. This immediate skin-to-skin contact has many benefits including helping to regulate baby's body temperature and heartbeat, keeping baby's blood sugars stable, and increasing the likelihood of successful breastfeeding. It also allows the baby to be 'colonised' by the same bacteria as the mother which, along with breastfeeding and vaginal birth, are thought to be important in the prevention of allergic diseases. These benefits are also important for premature babies, even if on oxygen or other support, and your midwife will help you to achieve this.

If there is a reason why mum can't (or doesn't want to) have skin-to-skin, then the option is equally open to dad. Dads can also bond with their baby in this way, and if you would like to, just take off your top and cuddle your baby to keep him or her warm and calm. Your baby will start to get to know you and to take in the world around them.

How do you wish to birth the placenta?

The third stage of labour can be a bit of an afterthought, as compared with the arrival of your baby, it isn't as exciting or interesting! The vast majority of women in the UK have a medically managed third stage, however, increasing numbers are beginning to really look at this choice, and its implications for the hour after birth.

It is always helpful to set a preference about the third stage for your birth plan. This does not mean that you can't change your mind on the day (you can change your mind about anything!) but having a preference is important so the birth partner can advocate your wishes at this point.

- **Medically managed stage.** This means the injection of a synthetic version of oxytocin to stimulate the uterus to contract. This is often followed by the midwife pulling on the umbilical cord/pushing on your tummy to help remove the placenta; you might be asked to change position after birth to accommodate this. Intervention does usually mean that the placenta is birthed more quickly than without. There is also a smaller risk of a postnatal bleed than with a natural third stage. However, there is a higher risk of parts of the placenta being retained, which could lead to infection or surgery to remove them.

- **Natural stage.** This means waiting for your body to produce its own oxytocin, to cause the uterus to contract of its own accord to expel the placenta. This can take up to an hour, but can be as little as five minutes! Keeping the environment conducive to oxytocin production will enable this to happen more quickly and safely. Keeping the umbilical cord unclamped until the placenta has been birthed is also beneficial to a natural third stage. The main benefit to a natural third stage is that you can focus on just being with your baby without any disruptions, and it can be a more comfortable experience.

When and if you clamp the cord?

Traditionally, clamping and cutting the umbilical cord was carried out by midwives within the first 30 seconds after the birth. However, evidence in the last few years has highlighted how this was not required or beneficial to the baby. 'Delayed cord clamping' means to delay the intervention of clamping the umbilical cord at the moment of birth.

After your baby has been birthed, as long as the cord is intact, the placenta continues to give the baby blood. In fact, up to a third of your baby's blood volume will be still in the cord and placenta at the time of their birth. Keeping your baby's cord unclamped allows your baby to still receive blood and oxygen from mum even though he or she has been born. This gives them a period of adjustment time as they get used to breathing for themselves.

Delaying the clamping of the cord also allows vital stem cells to be transferred to the baby. This allows for increased levels of iron to pass to baby, thereby lowering the risk of iron deficiency and anaemia, which can negatively affect brain development. It also means your baby's body does not have to work as hard in the early days to produce the blood volume left behind.

Up until a few years ago, it was believed that delayed cord clamping could cause jaundice in babies. However, it is now proven that babies are no more likely to become jaundiced by delaying cord clamping, and there is no relation between jaundice and the time of the cord being clamped.

If you wish to collect cord blood for storage or donation, the cord will need to be clamped immediately before it passes to your baby.

Some parents choose to not cut the umbilical cord at all, and leave baby attached to the placenta until the cord comes away naturally; this is known as a 'Lotus' birth. Some parents see this as a more natural period of transition for baby, allowing baby to let go gently of their mother's body, in their own time. It also can be a way of ensuring mum takes things very easily and keeps her baby close to her, as a baby with placenta still attached is harder to move around. So what are your choices?

- Immediate clamping of the cord.
- Delayed clamping of the cord for a set period of time – 1, 2, 3 minutes etc.
- Delaying the cord clamping until the cord has finished pulsating and transferring blood to your baby.
- Delaying the cord clamping until after the placenta has been delivered.
- Not cutting the cord at all; a Lotus birth (see above).

What happens to your placenta?

Did you know that you have choices about the placenta? If you wish to see it, or keep it, then these are options open to you. If you have no interest in the placenta, then that is fine, and the midwives will be happy to dispose of it for you. So what are your choices?

- To see your placenta and have a midwife explain it to you.
- To keep your placenta and do whatever you wish with it; some people choose to consume it, some people make jew-

ellery or art from it, and others choose to bury it in the garden as a special memory of the birth. If you want to keep it and do something with it, you can.

■ To have your placenta disposed of as medical waste.

Who cuts the cord?

If you have decided to have the cord clamped and cut, who do you want to do this? Many fathers enjoy the opportunity to do this, and see it as a rite into fatherhood, but who cuts the cord is a choice you can make. The mum, dad, another birth partner, or the midwife can all do this job.

If you are undecided, you can always keep the option open and see how you feel at the time. You could make a note on your birth plan that you would like to be given the option of cutting the cord so you have the discussion at the time.

Rest assured, neither mum nor baby will feel anything as the cord is cut, as there are no nerve endings in the cord. A pair of surgical scissors is used, and if you want to do it, the midwife will guide you, showing you exactly where to cut.

Vitamin K

One of the first medical treatments your baby will be offered is an injection of vitamin K. Vitamin K plays an important part in making blood clot. A very small number of newborn babies, about 1 in 10,000, have vitamin K deficiency bleeding (VKDB) and these babies don't have enough vitamin K. If a baby has a deficiency of vitamin K, he or she may spontaneously bruise or bleed within the first hours or days of birth.

What are your options when it comes to vitamin K? You can:

■ **Agree to a one-off injection of vitamin K for your baby after birth.** Medical experts agree that giving vitamin K by injection is the most effective and efficient way of protecting babies from VKDB. This is because one injection is all that is needed, and it gives the baby immediate protection.

As with any injection though, it can be painful and leave a bruise.

- **Have the vitamin k administered orally**. This is given to your baby over several doses, rather than injected as one large dose. Giving vitamin K by mouth is as effective at preventing VKDB, provided that the three doses are given when, and as they should be. This way means no painful injection for your baby, and smaller doses being given at a time.

- **Decline vitamin K being given to your baby.** Some parents decide that the likelihood of their baby being at risk of being vitamin k deficient are small. If your baby has had a straight-forward birth without any physical trauma such as forceps or ventouse, you may also decide that the likelihood of life-threatening bleeding is also minimal.

Whether or not you decide to give vitamin K to your baby, and how, you should make sure that you always report any unexplained bleeding to your doctor or midwife immediately.

CHAPTER 21

Home as a family

However your birth went, you are both likely to feel a little delicate at parts in the first few days. You may both be more tired than usual, or have moments of emotion. For mum, your body will feel different, you may have some soreness, or other physical changes to work through. So don't rush to be 'back to normal'; give yourself time to readjust.

Hers

Physical changes after birth
Your body will look different in the days after you have given birth, it is helpful to be aware of this so that you feel more comfortable and accepting of the changes in those first few days, weeks and months. They are a normal part of motherhood, and nothing to be ashamed about, and how your body looks in the first few days after motherhood is not how it will stay.

It is normal that in the days after birth, your tummy will be looser, after all your body grew to accommodate your baby and now they are no longer in there. Some mums describe their tummies as a 'deflated soufflé' after birth! You are likely to need to continue wearing maternity clothes for a while, but your tummy shape will continue to keep changing in the first days and weeks after birth as it readjusts.

You may also notice that you have stretch marks on your tummy, thighs, bottom or breasts. Like your tummy, these will change over time and are likely to fade.

If you developed a linea nigra (the dark line that runs down the middle of the tummy) during pregnancy, this is likely to remain for a while after birth, but will gradually fade.

Your breasts may be bigger, with more visible veins, and they may leak as your milk supply adjusts. As your breasts change shape and size, a good bra will help you cope with any backache or tenderness.

You may find that you start losing hair; during pregnancy increased levels of estrogen encouraged it to grow thicker, but as levels after birth fall, some of the extra hair naturally falls out.

You may need to wee more often, and experience night sweats, which are just your body's ways of getting rid of the extra water you retained during pregnancy.

About 20 per cent of mums experience constipation after giving birth, and it is not unusual not to poo for a couple of days. The digestive system slows down dramatically during labour, and it can take a little while to readjust back. Be prepared that midwives will ask you after each visit to the loo if you have opened your bowels, to check you are not uncomfortably constipated. If you are, let them know, so they can help.

If you had stitches or feel sore, it is normal to feel anxious about going to the toilet. Be assured that pooing is not likely to hurt, damage any stitches, or make any tears bigger. Feeling worried can make us physically tense, which may make it harder to go, so use any skills to relax that you have learnt (they are not just for labour!). Drink lots of water to help keep the poo soft.

When you go for a wee, the urine can cause any stitches to sting. If you find this makes going for a wee painful, try pouring warm water over the area to dilute your urine and wash it away from the area quickly. You can wee in the shower or bath too.

If you have a caesarean scar, keep comfortable by choosing pants which have a waistband that sit well above your stitches.

Your uterus contracts back to its pre-pregnancy size in the first days after birth, and you may experience 'after-pains' as this happens. These tend to be strongest during breastfeeding, and can range from minor discomfort to strong pains. Many women find they get stronger after each birth they have. Try using breathing practice or relaxation techniques to cope with them, but if they are very painful, talk to your midwife about painkillers.

You will experience blood loss ('lochia') after birth, which is like a very heavy period. This can last for anything up to six weeks after birth, and will change colour during that time. Lochia can also contain mucus and placenta tissue, so it is normal that you may see some small clots or lumps. The midwife and health visitor will ask you about your lochia, and if you have any concerns about it, just mention it. If you pass anything you are concerned about, keep it to show them.

How do you feel?

Having a baby is a life-changing experience, so in addition to all the physical changes you experience in the first days after birth, there may be a lot of emotional ones. Feelings of happiness, joy, pride, protectiveness, anxiety, worry... You may also have feelings of sadness if there were difficulties or trauma during your birth, or if you hoping or expecting a different gender. These mixed feelings are completely normal, so try not to be too hard on yourself for any 'negative' feelings in these early days. You are undergoing a huge life change and it takes time for everything to settle down.

Around 80 per cent of mums experience 'baby blues', which can make you feel emotional or irritable, cause you to burst into tears, or leave you feeling down or anxious. Baby blues is a short-lived experience caused largely by hormonal changes, and usually passes by the time your baby is two weeks old. However, if you find it doesn't, talk to your partner and midwife, health visitor or doctor, in case you need some support with postnatal depression (PND).

Try not to have too many expectations about how you will feel, or 'should' feel, in those first days as a family. Give yourself time to adjust to becoming a parent. Even if this is not your first baby, every baby brings with them a change to your life. Focus on one day at a time, rather than becoming overwhelmed about everything. Your baby will change day by day, and taking things as they come, rather than worrying about the possibilities, is kinder to you.

His

Babies are tiny, but their impact is huge. You will notice changes in your partner, your home environment, your day to day life, and of course, yourself, once your baby has arrived.

How do you feel?
How you feel can change several times in the course of the day: love, fear, happiness, awe, worry, guilt, security, tiredness, jealousy, resentment, pride, loss, protectiveness... You may have days when you want to escape from all the noise and changes and be on your own for a little while. These feelings are totally normal.

If you feel the need for a change of scene and some alone time, make it quick and if possible, useful! Pop out, bringing something home which is needed (dinner or a nice lunch is a good one), and something nice for your partner to show you were still thinking of her while you were out. Why not consider, if she feels up to it, all going out somewhere together. Even a short trip out for a coffee, or to feed the ducks, can help you all feel more refreshed.

What is helpful to realise is that your partner is going through her own range of profound feelings too. This isn't to minimise how you are feeling, but to realise that you are not alone. As her body adjusts to not being pregnant any more, your partner undergoes a series of hormonal changes that can have a very strong impact on her emotions and mood. In addition, she may feel physically sore and tired, dealing with a range of challenging physical symptoms that can have an impact on how she is feeling.

Your partner may not always want to tell you her feelings, as she may worry that they reflect badly on her, or suggest that she is not coping with being a mum. Just try to be aware that however you may feel in those early days, it can be a magnified experience for your partner. Your support is so important. Give your partner the opportunity to talk to you about how she feels, and encourage her to talk to you if you are worried about how she is coping emotionally.

Your role of advocate and protector are not over now that baby is here, of course. You need to think about protecting the environment around your partner, to allow her to recover and to encourage family bonding. This includes being gate-keeper to visitors, preparing meals and taking care of the housework – these things are all crucial.

If people feel the need to give their opinion on how you have chosen to birth, feed, care, carry your baby, etc. you can act as 'protector' for your family. Thank them politely for the input, but say that you are doing this your own way and you are sure they can respect that. Then change the subject! Make sure your partner never feels 'outnumbered', and never undermine her by disagreeing with her in front of visitors. Back her up, and then discuss it again later together in privacy, if appropriate. You are a team, and that means working together.

Going back to work

It is important to consider how your partner might feel when you return back to work. It is not unusual for some women to feel isolated or even abandoned on some level, as it goes from working together as a new family unit, a team, to suddenly being left on her own. If she has had difficulties feeding, is still sore or low, or baby is unsettled a lot of the time, it can magnify these anxious feelings. Of course, all people are different, and there will also be women who do not feel this way at all – but talking to your partner to find out how she feels, and how things have been each day is important. This way if things are not working out, you can then work together to find a way forwards.

When and if you do go back to work, make time to call your partner to ask her how she is doing, especially on the first day on her own. Show her that you care and you are thinking about them both. Arrange to pick up a takeaway or to do the cooking when you get home, and if you can, take her a little something home, even if it is just a bar of her favourite choco-late. All of these things can help to show that you do care and support her, even if you cannot always be there. By staying in touch and finding out what is happening in your absence, you will also feel more involved, which can help alleviate any sad-ness you might be feeling too.

When you come home on an evening from work, make the first hour of the day your time with baby while mum has some time to herself to have a bath or whatever she wants to do. It will give you that quality time with your little one which you have missed during the day, as well as giving your partner some space of her own.

On your days off, ask your partner whether she wants to stay in and relax or whether she would like to go out somewhere. New mums can feel pretty isolated once their partners have gone back to work, especially if they are not yet confident going out on their own, or are unable to drive themselves following a caesarean birth.

Get Together

Those first days after your baby arrives are a crucial time for spending time together as a new family getting to know each other, as well as time to rest and recover, and to learn about your new baby and work out what you are doing. Giving yourselves time to settle into being a family and just enjoying your baby is important and beneficial, but many new parents also want to balance this with introducing their baby to family and friends and not feeling too isolated from the world!

There are different choices you can make, and as with all parenting decisions, it comes down to your personal preferences. Try to focus on what feels right for you, rather than what you 'should' do or is expected of you. This is your baby and if you want to see people, see them! If you would rather not just yet, then don't!

Talk to each other about how you both feel about visitors before your baby arrives, but also revisit this discussion once baby has arrived as feelings can change.

Some of the possible options you could consider together for those first days and weeks include:

■ **Baby mooning.** Increasing numbers of new parents are now choosing to 'babymoon'. This means just being with their baby for a week or so. This means no visitors, just time dedicated to being together as a new family. This can mean lots of time for cuddles, skin-to-skin holding, and learning about your baby. Days can be spent in pyjamas at a slow pace, with minimal external demands. If mum is learning to breastfeed, it can be easier to not have to worry about doing it in front of other people, or feeling like she has to leave the room in her own home. The privacy of a babymoon allows space and time to learn and practise. For dads on paternity leave, the time will fly by, and baby mooning allows you the maximum time for bonding. This time when you get to know each other is precious and important, whether this is your first baby or your fifth. It can be awkward asking people to give you space and to wait before visiting, but it is only for a short while, and friends and family should understand that your needs as a new family have to come first.

- **Restrict visiting.** If you would like to receive some visitors, then arrange it so that it will not cause additional stress. Make sure that all visitors agree a date and time for their visit with you in advance. You could also request that they call before setting off to visit to make sure it is still convenient. If you do not want to be disturbed by unexpected visitors, then take control. Put a note on the door saying you are all sleeping today and do not want to be disturbed. Unplug the phone or change the answer machine message to say you are all fine, and to leave a message so you can call back at a convenient time.

- **Have a plan!** Discuss together how you both want to handle visitors, who you will allow over in those first couple of weeks, and for how long.

- **Dad the gatekeeper.** Dad acting as 'gatekeeper' can be a way to have all the visitors you want, with a safety net. You can agree that it is dad's role to get rid of them, if or when, mum feels she has had enough. Visitors can be very tiring, and if mum wants to have a nap, to feed baby in peace, or has just had enough, it can be awkward if others don't realise. You could agree a code word or phrase in advance, and if mum uses it in conversation, dad knows it is his cue to encourage the visitors to leave! This could be a phrase like: 'Would you mind getting me a glass of milk?' or whatever you like. This can make having visitors over feel much easier, as it gives you a way of communicating how you feel and what you need, without having to let everyone know.

- **Added benefit.** If a visitor offers to bring something with them, take them up on it! Ask them to bring lunch or dinner so you have one less meal to worry about, and you won't be expected to prepare food for large numbers of people. It might sound a bit cheeky, but people are usually happy to be able to help.

- **Choose who handles your baby.** Just because you have visitors does not mean you have to pass around your baby. If you want to keep your baby in your arms, then that is absolutely fine, and there are lots of benefits to you both in that. If you are happy to pass baby around for cuddles, then that's fine too. If you would prefer any visitors with a cold to not hold your baby, then it is perfectly acceptable to say so; suggest that they hold them next time.

Conclusion

We hope you have enjoyed reading our book, and that you find it a helpful tool to support you both as you go through pregnancy, birth, and those first early days together.

The book is really designed to be a starting point, so reaching the end of it is really the beginning of what comes next: your own discussions, choices, plans and possibilities.

Hopefully you will feel the book has given you both some understanding of what your partner might be feeling, experiencing or thinking about. Being able to put yourself into your partner's shoes, can help ease potential misunderstanding. At a time when we feel like life is changing all around us, when sleep deprived, trying to learn new skills, and with well-intentioned friends, family and professionals trying to tell you what to do, all couples come under a little strain. Any of this makes us more prone to arguing and bickering. As we say constantly throughout the book, the key is communication! Talk to each other about what is going on, and more importantly, listen to each other. Just because you might not feel the way your partner does, or you might disagree, doesn't make how they feel any less important or real. Being heard and reassured is an important part of processing feelings.

Don't feel you always have to 'solve' the concerns of your partner; it may not be possible or even what he or she wants.

Focus on how you can go forward, working together for the best interests of your own unique family, rather than worrying about choices other parents are making for theirs. Keep reading, keep researching. If you are going to use internet forums, remember that other people love to share and direct based on their own experiences, but you need to find what is right for you, in your own circumstances. Competitive parenting is unnecessary and largely unhelpful, as your pregnancy, birth and baby are unique.

Pregnancy is the ideal time to start the practice of working as a team, well before labour or before your baby arrives. If you can, invest time, effort and maybe even some finances into preparing for your birth; they do make a difference. If you want to learn more about some of the skills and techniques in this book with trained facilitators, visit The Natal Family website to find your nearest antenatal teacher and classes.

This is a time in your lives that can bring some of the most enjoyable experiences you will ever have. There will also be experiences that can grow your closeness as a couple and a family. We wish you all the best on your new journey together into parenthood.

Steph & Dean
Co-founders, The Natal Family

Useful Resources

MummyNatal www.mummynatal.co.uk

Our UK based antenatal classes for mums, covering a range of labour and birth skills, including breathing practice, birth ball techniques, relaxation and meditation.

Also available are birth workshops for couples, a great accompaniment to this book!

DaddyNatal www.daddynatal.co.uk

Our website for dads, here you will also be able to access DaddyNatal Online – our award winning antenatal classes for men from the comfort of your living room.

BabyNatal www.babynatal.co.uk

Our UK based antenatal classes for parents, focused on what you need to know about caring for your baby and parenting choices. From practical baby care skills such as bathing and winding, to first aid for babies, or developmental baby massage, our classes help you focus on learning the skills, information and choices as a parent.

Dad Info www.dad.info

A one-stop resource for life as a dad.

Kicks Count www.kickscount.org.uk

A charity providing information and support on the importance of baby's movements in pregnancy.

Birth Choice UK www.birthchoiceuk.com

A useful resource for comparing the maternity statistics of different birth places in the UK.

Birth Rights www.birthrights.org.uk

Provides legal information relating to women, families and birth.

Acknowledgements

Thanks have to go to Random House, for being so excited about the concept of this book, and working with us in the early stages to develop the idea.

A huge thanks have to go to Phil and Debbie at Slumberoo, and the team at Boba, for all their support and partnership and helping our classes reach more parents around the UK. They have been instrumental in enabling us to explore the practice and benefits of baby wearing with new and expectant parents.

Thank you to all teachers of The Natal Family – for the work you do with parents across the country, and the support you give to raise awareness of resources like this book. Thank you for your patience with us while it was being written – we hope it will be a useful resource for you as well as the parents you work with.

And finally thank you to all the friends, colleagues and clients, who continue to support us, our family and the work we do.

Index